Healing Toolbox Plus

■ ■ ■

A to Z Workshop

By Prince Handley

University of Excellence Press

Copyright © 2016 by Prince Handley
Revised 2018
All Rights Reserved.

ISBN-13: 978-0692774359
ISBN-10: 0692774351

UNIVERSITY OF EXCELLENCE PRESS
San Diego ▉ London ▉ Tel Aviv

Second Edition

✠

The only Healing Resource you need!

TABLE OF CONTENTS

FOREWORD

Several MIRACLE testimonies have been received as a result of the book, **Health and Healing Complete Guide to Wholeness**. Many people were made aware of their right to BOTH divine healing AND divine health ... plus learned HOW to appropriate the same via different methods described in the book.

The purpose of this book is to present "case–by–case" **specific** conditions (physical, mental and emotional) from which the reader may draw scriptural help, with a "tailored" plan of attack for each.

From **anxiety and panic attacks** to **mental disease and depression** ... from **bipolar disorder** to **cancer** ... from **jaw and head pain** to **relationships**. That's WHY we have chosen the title, **Healing Toolbox Plus: A to Z Workshop**. Different conditions—various—numerous subjects are covered for the reader. This book is truly an encyclopedia of—*scriptural*—divine healing and health.

Interweaved—at strategic places—throughout the book are chapters to BOTH build your faith for healing AND provide additional "tools" for healing.

Now ... be healed ... and then YOU go heal others!

Healing Toolbox Plus

■ ■ ■

A to Z Workshop

FOUR THINGS TO KNOW

■ You do not have to be sick.

■ God promises your healing.

■ God wants you to be healed.

■ God provided for the healing.

~ CHAPTER ONE ~

HEALING FROM FEAR AND SHAME

Fear and shame are two weapons your enemy, Satan, will use against you to cause oppression, rejection, physical or mental sickness, and lack of production in your life. In this chapter we will discuss HOW to be healed—and delivered permanently—from both fear and shame!

There is an old saying, *"You are as others see you."* The devil knows if you have FEAR in your heart. If you do, ask God to help you. Ask him to take the fear away. King David said, *"What time I am afraid, I will trust in thee (the LORD)."* (Psalm 56:3) Go to the Word of God and RECEIVE BY FAITH the power promised in the scriptures, such as: *"For God has not given us the spirit of fear; but of power, and of love, and of a sound mind."* (2 Timothy 1:7)

Fear is a spirit; therefore, you must speak to it. God is love and He is spirit. Love is stronger than fear. Perfect love casts out fear. *"There is no fear in love;*

8

but perfect love casts out fear: because fear has torment. He that fears is not made perfect in love." (1 John 4:18)

If you are afraid of someone, ask God to give you His love for them. You can bind fear in the name of Yeshua (Jesus) , and cast it away from you.

Command fear to leave, and use the name of Jesus against it. Speak (declare) the BLOOD of Messiah against it. It is your responsibility to overcome fear.

Serious cases of fear require four (4) steps:

> **1.** A stayed (fixed) mind. You are NOT going to quit until you eliminate fear totally from your life.
>
> **2.** Confession of God's Word (1 John 4:18; James 4:7; 2 Timothy 1:7).
>
> **3.** A step of faith ... action. Speak to fear and take authority over it.
>
> **4.** Intercession and spiritual warfare (for others or one's self).

IMPORTANT: The reason for this attack of fear is to get you to STOP action!

The enemy's chief concern is that you STOP doing what you are currently involved in doing. You have been TOO SUCCESSFUL; also, your plans for future endeavors are causing him to freak out. The devil is the most frustrated person in the world today; he knows that his time is running out. When the fullness of the Goyim (Gentiles) takes place, then all Israel (the nation as a whole) will be saved. (Romans 11)

SunTzu, in his book, *The Art of War*, says: *"Every battle is won before it is fought."* How true in spiritual warfare: even the whole war is won because of the victory of our Lord Jesus, the Messiah. His death, burial, and resurrection conquered the enemy and bought our freedom and eternal life. **We take ACTION on that victory by appropriating it in faith as we move forward**.

Another weapon in the arsenal of the enemy, in addition to fear, is shame. **The enemy will try to attack you with imposed shame**.

Lots of times, the enemy will attack even seasoned warriors with **imposed shame from family members or friends** as a result of some fault or failure from the past.

There are **many examples of shame experienced by people of God in the Bible**. We are NOT perfect: that's why we need a Savior! Abraham (the same as) sold his wife two times. Moses killed a man in anger. David committed adultery and murder. Peter denied Messiah three times in one night. We see that Adam's shame was manifested in hiding.

In Revelation 3:18, Yeshua admonished the synagogue at Laodicea to *"Buy of me white raiment, that you may be clothed, [so] that the shame of your nakedness does not appear."*

There are several types of shame:

- Adamic shame

- Inherited shame

- Actual shame

- Imposed shame

Every one of these types of shame may be remitted, or canceled, by the atonement of Messiah. **The BLOOD Yeshua shed on the cross-stake paid for you and your sins, and provides healing for shame.**

The verdict of guilt, whether real or imagined, is shame. It may be something inherited **from Adam** (who brought sin into the world as the federal head of the race); or it may be something inherited **from ancestral, or family lines.** It may be actual shame, resulting **from an action** you have initiated. And, **it may be psychological shame**—real or false shame—**that people or demon spirits have tried to impose upon you,** resulting in oppression, rejection, physical or mental sickness, and lack of production.

Messiah Yeshua bore your shame. Hebrews 12:2 in the Brit Chadashah (New Testament) tells us that our Lord Yeshua despised the shame of the cross-stake and his nakedness thereon, but went through **it because of the JOY set before Him:** that is,Hhe saw YOU able to be made whole and to know God, with your sins forgiven and having eternal life, as the result of His sacrifice. Yeshua despised shame, and He despises it in YOUR life. He died for YOU so that **you do NOT have to carry shame. He carried it for YOU!**

Yeshua (Jesus) is alive to remit guilt and its resultant shame from your life today. You can appropriate the healing in His shed BLOOD for you by calling on Him today. Pray and ask Jesus to deliver you. If you are not sure you know Him, then pray this prayer.

"God of Abraham, Isaac, and Jacob, if Jesus is really my Messiah, then reveal Him to me."

If God reveals Him to you, then receive Him and live for Him. **Ask God what He wants you to do with your life!**

You can get back up because He got back up! **The Messiah has need of you in these last days.**

~ CHAPTER TWO ~
HEALING OF UNBELIEF
DO YOU REALLY WANT TO BE HEALED?

More people are kept from being healed and made whole **by unbelief** than are those who just do NOT know that healing belongs to them.

Healing is a both a **right** and a **privilege**.

If we know Yeshua the Messiah, then it is **our right to be healed**. Both the Tanakh (the Jewish Old Testament) and the Brit Chadashah (the Jewish New Testament) tell us that **healing is in the Atonement**. The *Torah* (the five Books of Moses) tells us:

> *"For the life of the flesh is in the blood: and I have given it to you upon the altar to make an atonement for your souls: for it is the blood that makes an atonement for the soul."* (Leviticus 17:11)

The word "**atonement**" from the Hebrew "**kaphar**" means "**to cover, to cancel, to cleanse, to forgive, to purge away**."

Isaiah the prophet, 750 years **before** Messiah Yeshua came to earth, prophesied:

> "Surely he has borne our **sicknesses** and **diseases** [Hebrew: **choli**], and carried away our **pains** [Hebrew: **macob**]: yet we did esteem him stricken, smitten of God, and afflicted.
>
> But he was wounded for our **sin, rebellion, and trespasses** [Hebrew: **pesha**], he was bruised for our iniquities: the chastisement of our peace was upon him; and **with his stripes we are healed**.
>
> All we like sheep have gone astray; we have turned every one to his own way; and the LORD has **laid on him** the iniquity of us all." (Tanakh: Isaiah 53:4-6)

I have included the original Hebrew root words in the passage because in the English Bible, the sense has been watered down. **Why?** The translators who translated from Hebrew into English did NOT believe in divine healing—*like many today*—and so did not believe that healing was included in the Atonement.

When Messiah Yeshua was on earth 750 years **after** Isaiah, he fulfilled this prophecy. In the Brit Chadashah (the Hebrew New Testament) we read:

> *"When the evening came, they brought unto him many that were possessed with demons; and he* ***cast out the spirits with his word****, and* ***healed all that were sick****: so that it might be* ***fulfilled which was spoken by Isaiah the prophet****, saying,* ***Himself took our infirmities, and bare our sicknesses.****"* (Matthew 8:16-17)

Healing—spiritual, mental, and physical—is included in the Atonement. When Messiah shed His holy sinless BLOOD, it was the **one-time final supreme sacrifice**: payment for your sins and mine. He was the spotless lamb of God who was sacrificed in our place.

Messiah Yeshua took our sins upon himself on the cross stake and healed the separation between God and man. Adam, the first man who lived, caused that separation in the Garden of Eden. Adam separated us from God. **Separation from God cuts us off from God's life.** When we are separated from the life of God, the result is spiritual death. **Spiritual death produces physical death.** God sent His Son, Yeshua, to heal the separation

16

and **connect us with the life source of God** so our spirits could be reborn eternally, and our bodies could have healing life available up until it is time for us to leave this earth.

By one man [Adam] sin came into the world, and death by sin.

By one man [Messiah] many shall be made righteous (have right standing with God).

> *"For as by the disobedience of one man [Adam] many were made sinners, so by the obedience of one [Messiah] shall many be made righteous."*

Healing belongs to you! Yeshua has connected you with the life source of God. **Messiah is your atonement: your covering**. If you are NOT sure that God sent His Son to earth to pay for your sins, then pray this prayer:

> *"God of Abraham, Isaac, and Jacob, if Yeshua (Jesus) is really your Son ... and if He is really my Messiah ... then reveal Him to me. **I ask you to heal me today**. Please forgive my sins. I will serve you the rest of my life."*

You're going to have a wonderful future, my friend!

~ CHAPTER THREE ~
HEALING THROUGH RELEASE

I want to talk to you in this chapter about healing through release, or **healing through forgiveness**.

Notice, forgiveness is associated with being tenderhearted. Forgiveness will also keep you tenderhearted. It prevents your heart (your emotions and spirit) from being hardened. If God has forgiven us for ALL the things we have done, how can we NOT forgive someone for what they have done, no matter how insidious or pernicious it may have been ... especially in the LIGHT of eternity.

One time I was going to the post office to post a ministry mail out. While I was on my way, **I was having a hard time forgiving someone**. As I entered the parking lot at the post office, **the LORD said to me**: *"Why are you letting that person rob you out of blessings? Why are you letting them bind you? Why are you letting them keep your prayers from being answered? Why are you letting* *them hinder you by your not forgiving them? Release them so I can bless you!"*

All of a sudden, the LIGHT came on in both my spirit and my mind. I said, *"God, I am NOT going to let them rob me out of blessings any more. They have already caused me enough grief and trouble. I forgive them right now in the name of Yeshua. I release them into your hands."*

Immediately the LORD flooded my soul with joy. The Bible tells us: *"Vengeance belongs to me; I will repay, says the Lord."*

One trick of the devil is to cause people to do things wrong to you, or to lie about you (or, lie to you), or to wound you emotionally. In a later chapter we will discuss **Healing of Wounds**.

There is a strategy behind the attacks of Satan. One reason for his attacks as he uses other people (sometimes a child of God) is to get you angry and emotionally disturbed. Even if you are not manifesting external responses, the devil knows that if you are disturbed internally, and harbor a spirit of unforgiveness, it will keep you from the blessings of God. That is just ONE of the reasons he likes to cause you trouble.

The scripture admonishes us to *"Be angry, and do not sin. Do not let the sun go down on your wrath, neither give **place** to the devil."* (Ephesians 4:27) The original Greek word for **place** here used is the word **topos**, which means: **a place to occupy, (or, as a military term, a place from which to attack you)**. Do NOT give the devil an opportunity to cause you to hate those who injure you, or to cause you to take revenge, or to silently harbor ill feelings and unforgiveness.

When I was a little boy, my sister and I shared the same bedroom. One day we had an argument (probably many days!). But that particular night as I was in my bed I was angry at my sister for some reason. Before I could go to sleep, she spoke to me from her bed on the other side of the room and said, *"Daddy always taught us never to go to bed mad."* So we made up. That is very good advice, and even though I did not realize it them, was scriptural: *"Do not let the sun go down on your wrath."*

My friend, God loves you so much, and He wants to BLESS you. Do not let the enemy of God, and your enemy (the devil), trick you into being bound by another person or people. If you have been wronged, or maybe lied about with absolutely no merit to the accusation, forgive. **Why would you let them bother you anymore?** Why would you let them bind you? Why would you let them rob you out of blessings? **Release them so God can bless you**.

Picture yourself with a chain or rope tied to that person or those people who have wronged you. **Forgive them and the chains and ropes - your chains and ropes - will drop off**. Give NO place - no location for military operations against you – to the devil.

You will not only experience release for yourself, but a freedom in your spirit, and the the dove of the Spirit of God—the Ruach Elohim—will flood your soul. Blessings will begin to abound.

"And be kind to one another, tenderhearted, forgiving each other, just as God also in Messiah forgave you." (Ephesians 4:32)

I trust this teaching will help you.

~ CHAPTER FOUR ~
HEALING FROM CONFUSION

There is lots of confusion today about sickness and disease ... even about natural disasters like hurricanes, tsunamis, and earthquakes. The confusion lies in the "cause" of such things. Even the insurance companies try to "opt out" of liability for such things as "natural disasters" which they refer to in their policy exclusions as "acts of God."

Even in some synagogues and churches it is being taught that everything that comes your way is God's will for you and (in particular) that if you are suffering sickness or disease, God is trying to teach you something. However, it is best to let the Word of God speak for itself. **In the Torah we see in Deuteronomy Chapter 28 that sickness and disease is a curse ... NOT a blessing.**

When Messiah Yeshua was on earth, He said, *"If you have seen me, you have seen the Father."* In other words, you have seen the Father's nature. If you read the Brit Chadashah (the Hebrew New Testament), you will quickly see that Yeshua (Jesus) never made anyone sick. As in the Torah, we see that disobedience CAN cause the curse of sickness and disease. Also, because of Adam's (original) sin in the Garden of Eden, man was separated from God. **When man was separated from God, he was separated from the life source.**

This is WHY God sent His Son to earth, to HEAL the separation between God and man. The atonement of Yeshua, God's Son, on the cross stake paid for our sins … and purchased our healing (spiritual, mental, and physical) by His BLOOD that was shed. Messiah Yeshua's blood contained the life of God. Messiah was born of a virgin, and therefore His blood did NOT contain the sinful blood from Adam's seed line. His blood was the one-time FINAL payment for our sins, and brought us into right standing (or, righteousness) with God, whereby we have wholeness when we exercise our faith in Messiah's sacrifice for us.

We see from the scriptures how sickness and disease is from the Evil One, and NOT from the Father God. Messiah NEVER refused healing to anyone. *"How God anointed Yeshua (Jesus) of Nazareth who went about doing good, and healing ALL that were oppressed of the devil, for God was with Him."* (Brit Chadashah: Acts 10:38)

*"And Yeshua went about all the cities and villages, teaching in their synagogues, and preaching the gospel of the kingdom, and healing **every sickness** and **every disease** among the people."* (Brit Chadashah: Mattiyahu [Matthew] 9:35)

Sickness and disease are from the devil. Healing and health are from God. Don't be confused about the source(s) of sickness and disease ... even about natural disasters like hurricanes, tsunamis, and earthquakes. I'll give you something to help you the rest of your life. **Put the devil on the left side and Messiah on the right side** with this verse from John 10:10 in the Hebrew New Testament. Yeshua said, *"The thief (the devil) comes to steal, to kill, and to destroy; but I (Messiah) have come that you might have life, and have it more abundantly."* Now you will be able to discern where things have their source; how and why they happen.

If you need healing today, or if you need miracles—real miracles—then pray this prayer:

"Father in Heaven, I ask you to reveal to me if Yeshua (Jesus) is my Messiah. I need healing; I need a miracle. Please heal me. In Jesus' name I pray. Amen."

I know this teaching will help you. Live a full life helping others!

~ CHAPTER FIVE ~
THE LORD'S HEALING NATURE
NEVER CHANGES

Psalm 103 gives us a powerful promise from God to any and ALL who may be suffering from disease: **spiritual, physical, or mental**.

"Bless the LORD, O my soul: and all that is within me, bless his holy name.

Bless the LORD, O my soul, and forget not all his benefits:

Who forgives all your iniquities [sins]; who HEALS ALL YOUR DISEASES." – Psalm 103:1-3

God's nature never changes. The **same** healing nature of YHWH that was revealed in the Tanach (the Old Testament of the Holy Bible) is revealed in the Brit Chadashah (the New Testament). **His nature is the same today as it was yesterday**.

In the Old Testament, God said, *"For I am the LORD, I change not."* In the New Testament we read, *"Yeshua the Messiah is the same yesterday, and today, and forever."* – Malachi 3:6 and Hebrews

Yeshua displayed the healing nature of God, Yeshua said, *"He who has seen me has seen the Father."* – Yochanan / John 14:9

Yeshua's nature is God's nature. **He never refused healing to anyone!** Yeshua is God!

*"And Yeshua went about all the cities and villages, teaching in their synagogues, and preaching the gospel [good news] of the kingdom, and **healing EVERY disease and every sickness** among the people."*

– Matthew 9:35

Yeshua came to earth to heal us, to make us whole ... to restore to health: spiritually, physically, and mentally. He came to **buy back** what Adam, the first man who ever lived, lost. In the garden of Eden, Adam sinned against God by disobeying him. God had commanded Adam:

28

"Of every tree of the garden you may freely eat. But of the tree of the knowledge of good and evil, you shall not eat of it; for in the day you shall eat of it you shall surely die." – TORAH: Genesis 2:16-17

Satan, the devil, lied to Eve, Adam's wife, saying, "You shall not surely die." But Eve, like many people today, did not realize that **REAL death is spiritual! Physical death (when your body dies) is merely a result of "spiritual" death. To be spiritually dead does not mean you do not exist; it simply means you exist, but that you are SEPARATED from God: joined to Satan!**

From one act of disobedience by Adam, sin entered into the world, so that spiritual death passed through the bloodline to ALL men ... resulting in physical death.

"Wherefore, as by one man (Adam) sin entered into the world, and death by sin; so death passed upon ALL men, for all have sinned." – Romans 5:12

This "spiritual" death—SEPARATION FROM GOD—which produced physical sickness and disease, and the death of the body, HAD TO BE HEALED! **This** is why God sent his only Son, Jesus the Messiah, to earth.

You can be healed today ... **NOW** ... by calling on the name of the LORD: Who forgives **all** your sins, and Who heals **all** your diseases. (Psalm 103:3)

The LORD's healing nature never changes. It is God's will to heal you!

~ CHAPTER SIX ~

HEALING FOR ALL SICKNESS
AND DISEASE

In order to receive help, you must first realize you have a need. But, this is NOT enough. You must also KNOW and be confident that there is a solution for your problem ... and that this solution—*the answer*—is attainable.

The answer must also be attainable by means of access. That is, can you interface with the answer (do you have a connection)? Is the source affordable? Is the solution legal? Is the help available? Is the resource or cure within a reasonable proximity?

Many people—if not most—are confused about the **origin** of sickness and disease and not only the WHERE (it came from) but the WHY (the purpose it serves, if any). Many people—if not most—have been taught that everything that happens to them in life is the will of God. However, IF sickness is the will of God for you, why does the Holy Bible say:

"Is any sick among you? Let him call for the elders of the church, and let them pray over him, anointing him with oil in the name of the Lord; and the prayer of faith shall save the sick and the Lord shall raise him up ..." (Brit Chadashah: James 5:14-150

If sickness is the will of God for you, then it is SIN for you to go to the doctor, or to take medicine, or to pray for healing, or to try to alleviate the condition by any means. Messiah Yeshua taught that human conditions evolve from either of two sources: Satan ... OR ... God.

"The thief [Satan, the devil] only comes to steal, to kill, and to destroy. I [Yeshua] came that they [the people on earth] may have life, and may have it abundantly." (Brit Chadashah: Yochanan 10:10)

If you know Messiah Yeshua personally, you do NOT have to be bound by sin, sickness, or disease. Because of the Edenic curse (which resulted from the first human being—Adam—who disobeyed God and sinned in the Garden of Eden), **you are going to face three (3) things in your lifetime: sin, sorrow, and death. "Three strikes and you're out!"** But, the Good News is that **if you know Messiah Yeshua personally—as**

your Lord—you can have victory over all three ...
PLUS eternal life.

The devil wants to steal from you, to kill you, and to destroy you ... but Yeshua (Jesus) wants to give you LIFE abundantly here on earth ... and in Heaven for eternity.

Sickness and disease are NOT the will of God for you. **You can be healed today.**

> *"Behold, I am the LORD, the God of **all flesh**: is there anything too hard for me?"* – Tanakh: Jeremiah 32:27

> *"God anointed Jesus of Nazareth with the Ruach ha Chodesh (the Holy Spirit) and with power; who went about doing good and **healing all** who were oppressed by the devil, for God was with him."* – Brit Chadashah: acts 10:38

> *"Yeshua ha Meshiach [Jesus the Anointed One] **is the same** yesterday, today, and forever."* – Brit Chadashah: Hebrews 13:8

> *"Praise the LORD, my soul! All that is within me, praise his holy name!*

*Praise the LORD, my soul, And **don't forget all his benefits: Who forgives all your sins; Who heals all your diseases; Who redeems your life from destruction."*** – Psalm 103-1-4

"For I, the LORD, do not change; *therefore you, sons of Yacov, are not consumed."* – Tanakh: Malachi 3:6

If you need healing today ... from sin, sickness, or disease ... the LORD is waiting to heal you right NOW. Ask Him. If you do not know Him, them pray this prayer:

"God of Abraham, Isaac, and Jacob, if Yeshua (Jesus) is really my Messiah, then reveal Him to me. I want to know Him personally as my Lord. Please forgive my sins and heal me. Help me to live for you here on earth and take me to Heaven to be with you when I die."

My friend, God wants the BEST for YOU. Now ... **you go help others!**

~ CHAPTER SEVEN ~
HEALING FROM CANCER

One of the most insidious diseases known to humankind is cancer. WHY? ... Because it brings fear with it. Just the name many times puts people into a psychological and emotional bondage that is hard for them to overcome both mentally and spiritually.

But if you believe God and believe His Holy Word, remember what is written: *"Behold, I am the LORD, the God of all flesh: is there any thing too hard for me?"* (Tanakh: Jeremiah 32:27) And let me direct you to a few of the chapters in this book:

Healing for All Sickness and Disease

How to Know that Healing is the Will of God

Healing of Unbelief

How to Be Healed (healing scriptures)

Let me first say that IF you have been diagnosed with cancer—no matter what kind—do NOT give up hope ...

35

and remember that FAITH is the **substance** of things for which you HOPE (Hebrews Chapter 11, verse 1). Faith is the evidence of things NOT seen. It's as simple as this: **you can CREATE (make) what you hope for from your faith!** Build your faith by reading and SPEAKING and believing what is written in the Word of God. Speak these scriptures aloud to yourself daily until they are strong in your inner man. You can find healing scriptures in the chapter, *Scriptures for Healing.*

Also, stay fit emotionally: walk, exercise, eat good food. **Tomatoes are believed to be one of the best cancer fighting foods available: heat them up to release the lycopene.** Lycopene is currently the most powerful antioxidant which has been measured in food. Other foods high in lycopene are:

> Guavas;
> Watermelon;
> Grapefruit;
> Dried parsley and basil;
> Persimmons;
> Asparagus;
> Liver;

Chili powder; and,

Red cabbage.

Pray and ask G-d if you are to undertake any medical treatment. There is nothing wrong with going to physicians or seeking medical help or advice. But what we should do is seek the LORD first to see what He wants us to do. He may want to heal us by His sovereign power, over a period of time, or instantly. Remember what happened to King Asa. In the 39th year of King Asa's rule, he was diseased in his feet until his disease was very critical. Yet, in his disease, he did not seek the Lord, but went to the physicians for help. He died two years later. [Tanakh: 2 Chronicles 16:11-13] Also if you are undergoing medical treatment. Pray and ask G-d to use the medications and/or treatment.

Never give up hope. Remember, the Holy Bible tells us: "And now continually enduring are these three: faith, hope, and love; but the greatest of these is love." Love is one of the greatest healing agents on earth. Conversely, hatred, bitterness and unforgiveness are the most damaging agents on earth. Study Hindrances to Healing and Wholeness (under the section **'Prayer**

and Proper Mental Attitude' in my book: *"Health and Healing: Complete Guide to Wholeness."*

If you are considering therapy of any kind you should also consider this: Which is MORE important for you: **Quality** of life? or, **Quantity** of life? If you desire QUALITY of life, then NO treatment may be your best option. If you desire QUANTITY of life, then therapy (including surgery, radiation, chemo therapy, Cyber Knife or Proton therapy) may be your option. However, realize that some chemical (or, hormonal) therapy such as ADT (Androgen Deprivation Therapy) may use chemical injections via shots **that can cause serious side effects**. You should search online support groups to find what people are experiencing from such medicines. Here is one online support group that is excellent: "Health Unlocked." Whichever option you decide upon ... just as the person who chooses to trust God with NO therapy ... **you should do what God leads YOU to do** ... and trust Him for your healing ... as well as health.

>>> CHECK OUT ADT DRUGS <<<

ADT drugs can have serious side effects. One such drug, Lupron, should be carefully considered before allowing any healthcare practitioner (MD's, Oncologists, Urologists included) to administer this medicine. If you do feel like your primary goal is "quantity" of life versus "quality" of life [you are just trying to extend your life], then perhaps you should only consider a one month (or, at the most 3 month) injection to see what the side effects are in YOU. If you have a 6 month injection you may have to wait from 8 months to 12 months for the side effects to wear off (depending upon your age and / or health).

In some cases health care professionals may use the trade names Lupron, Eligard, Lupron Depot, and Viadur when referring to the generic drug name Leuprolide. It is classifed as an "LHRH agonist."

***

Try to ENJOY life while you are believing God for your healing. Laughter, it is said, is the best ever medicine. It increases your endorphin levels, raises your immunity, lowers your cholesterol, releases muscular tension and even massages your internal organs. I heard about a man who cured himself of cancer by watching Laurel and Hardy movies.

Whenever we laugh we feel better about ourselves, our lives and everyone around us. It bonds us to our friends and work colleagues and instantly helps to relieve any emotional tension we're feeling. Watch some good old comedy films: Buster Keaton, Laurel and Hardy, The Three Stooges, Charles Chaplin, Fatty Arbuckle, and others.

NOTICE

One minute of laughter results in 24 hours of your immunity being increased. However, one minute of anger causes a six hour drop in your immunity.

There are some inexpensive ways to increase your immunity. Melatonin (3mg) is not only reported to be good for your sleep patterns, but also as an anti-oxidant to strengthen your immune system. Also, Vitamin C (50 to 100 mg) is reported to be good for fighting cancer and some say similar to chemotherapy.

There are certain foods you should avoid. There was a study at Rutger's University which found that the BOX which packaged cereal had more nutritional content than the cereal inside. Refined sugar is also NOT good to eat as it has no vitamins and no fibre; and, is reported to "feed" cancer.

Along with the lycopene type vegetables I mentioned above, fruit and berries are excellent foods. I usually make one or two fruit smoothies every day: bananas, black berries, blueberries, strawberries and sometimes mix vanilla or banana flavored protein powder in them. It is reported that 50 grams a day of nuts (I usually start my day with almonds) can add five years to your lifespan and can also strengthen your heart.

Some of the worst foods you can eat are cold cut (pre-packaged) meats with preservatives. They are carcinogenic and can cause cancer. The same goes with most "processed" foods. Also, try NOT to microwave too much (30 seconds probably is OK) as too long (more than 5 minutes) can destroy the protein value of food.

CHECK OUT IP-6

IP-6, inositol hexaphosphate, is a vitamin-like substance. It is found in animals and many plants, especially cereals, nuts, and legumes. It can also be made in a laboratory.

Some people use IP-6 to treat and prevent cancer, including prostate cancer, breast cancer, colon cancer, liver cancer, and blood cancers.

Researchers have been studying the role of IP-6 in cancer treatment and prevention since 1988. But, so far, there have been no studies in people with cancer. A book called *IP-6, Nature's Revolutionary Cancer-Fighter* by prominent IP-6 researcher Abulkalam M. Shamsuddin, MD, Ph.D, has popularized IP-6 as an anti-cancer tool.

IP-6 is also used for boosting the immune system, treating anemia, and preventing heart disease and kidney stones. In manufacturing, IP-6 is added to food to keep it from spoiling.

HOW IP-6 WORKS

IP-6 might help treat and prevent cancer by slowing down the production of cancer cells. It might also bind to certain minerals, decreasing the risk of colon cancer. IP-6 is also an antioxidant.

It's never too late to start being a good steward of what God has given you. Many people are good stewards (managers) of their finances, but miserable stewards of their body. What good is it to lay up finances for yourself if you are NOT going to live long enough to enjoy them. More importantly, what good is it even for you to be a good steward and lay up finances for the Kingdom of God if you are going to cut your life short by reason of ill health and only be able to produce for the Kingdom of God 80 years ... of 111?

I trust this teaching will encourage you to trust God and receive your healing, and then help you to become an instrument of healing for others in the future ... while YOU enjoy His prosperity to share with others and build His Kingdom.

OTHER RESOURCES

National Comprehensive Cancer Network

www.nccn.org

Phone 888-909-NCCN

American Cancer Society

www.cancer.org

Phone 800-ACS-2345

Prostate Cancer Foundation

www.pcf.org

Phone 800-757-CURE

~ CHAPTER EIGHT ~
HEALING FROM THE BONDAGE
OF SATAN: DELIVERANCE

Deliverance belongs to you! To "deliver" is to "set free". Yeshua (Jesus) said, *"And you shall know the truth, and the truth shall make you free."* (John 8:32)

If you know Messiah Yeshua as your LORD, NO demon, NO evil spirit can have you! Jesus said, *"If the Son therefore shall make you free, you shall be free indeed."* The Greek word here used for "indeed" (ontos) means "really, actually".

If you will study the Word of God, you will KNOW that Yeshua has set you FREE, and the devil cannot have you! Resist the devil with the Word of God. Speak God's Word to him and he will run away from you! James 4:7 tells us, *"Submit yourselves therefore to God. Resist the devil, and he will flee from you."*

To obtain FREEDOM in Messiah is to obtain freedom from Satan and all his demon spirits! You shall be FREE indeed!

Ask yourself the following questions:

Is Messiah Yeshua the LORD of my life?

Is there any unforgiveness in my heart?

Am I involved in, or have I been involved with -

Cults?

The occult, or occult practices?

Satanism or witchcraft (of any kind)?

Have I done or spoken evil to a minister or rabbi of the Good News of Messiah?

If the answers to #2, #3, or #4 above are "Yes", then do the following:

1. Pray to God and ask Him for forgiveness.

2. Renounce Satan: tell the devil that you no longer want anything to do with him or his works or workers.

Talk to the devil (renounce him) like this (command him):

> *"Satan, I renounce you and all your dark works and workers. In the name of Messiah Jesus who defeated you with His BLOOD and with His RESURRECTION, I command you to leave me. I belong to the LIVING Messiah Yeshua (Jesus). I take authority over you in the name of JESUS and cast you out of my life!"*

Note: Use this same prayer for your family!

3. Stay under the BLOOD of Messiah. If you can, find a good church or messianic synagogue which teaches the Good News of Messiah. and believes in healing and the gifts of the Holy Spirit. Read the Holy Bible and pray every day. Pray in tongues much to help build yourself up! Speak (declare) the BLOOD of Messiah over your life, your family, and your home every day.

4 Do NOT ally yourself closely with people who are involved in cults or the occult: such as tarot cards, ouija boards, seances, psychic phenomena, new-age meditation and the like. (You are still to love them and communicate Christ's Good News.) Read in

Deuteronomy 18:10-12in the Torah to see what God thinks about this!

The Bible says, *"The curse causeless shall not come."* You do NOT have to worry if people try to put curses on you **if you know Messiah Jesus!** Do NOT be afraid. Remember the old saying: *"Fear knocked at the door. Faith answered, and no one was there."*

~ CHAPTER NINE ~
HOW TO KNOW HEALING
IS THE WILL OF GOD

You need to know it is God's will to heal you. Not just God CAN heal you, but God WILL heal you! He wants to heal you and He PROMISES in His Word to heal you. His will is for you to fulfill the number of your days in HEALTH.

I want to talk to you in this chapter about *"Is Healing For Everyone?"* Or, another title would be *"How To Know It Is God's Will To Heal You."*

Healing is **still** the will of God as it was in the past. **It is God's will to heal ALL who have need of healing—and to fulfill the number of their days!** The greatest barrier to those who are seeking mental healing as well as physical healing is the uncertainty in their mind as to whether it is the will of God to heal everyone.

Nearly everyone believes that God heals some, but there is much in modern theology that keeps people from knowing what the Holy Bible teaches that **healing is for everyone.**

It's impossible to boldly claim by faith a blessing that were NOT SURE that God offers, because **the power of God can be claimed only when the will of God is known.** For example, concerning salvation, it would be nearly impossible to get someone to believe unto righteousness before you had fully convinced them that it is God's will to save them. **God wants to save people—and He wants to heal them!** He wants people to live in Heaven with Him: forever!

Faith begins where the will of God is known. If it is God's will to heal only some of those who need healing, then none have any basis for faith unless they have a special revelation that they are among the chosen ones. Faith must rest on the will of God alone and not on our desires and wishes. In this book I attempt to show WHY and HOW it is the will of God to heal—everyone!

Appropriating faith is not believing that God can, but that God will. Lots of God's people will tell you, *"Oh, I believe that God CAN heal me."* However, the WILL of God is what we want. Do they believe, *"Yes I believe that God WILL heal me."* Because of not knowing that healing is a redemptive privilege for **everyone**, most of those in our day, when asking God for healing, add to the end of their prayer the phrase, *"if it is your will."*

Among all those who sought healing from the Messiah Yeshua during His earthly ministry, we read of only one who had this kind of theology. That was the leper who said, *"Lord, IF you will, you can make me clean."* **The first thing Messiah Yeshua did was to correct the leper's theology by saying, "I will. You be clean."** Yeshua's "I will" cancelled the leper's "If." Adding to the leper's faith that Messiah COULD heal him, that He WOULD heal him!

The theology of this leper before Messiah enlightened him is almost universal today, because this part of the Good News of Messiah Yeshua is so seldom and fragmentarily preached. And we see from almost every conceivable angle throughout the scriptures there is no doctrine—no teaching—more clearly taught than that it **IS** God's will to heal ALL: everyone who has need of healing. And that they my fulfill the number of their days according to His promise(s).

Remember that all those who Yeshua called back from the dead were young people who had not lived out their fullness of years. **And in that very fact we may see Messiah's protest against premature death.** Of course we must not expect that the old shall be physically young, but **if the allotted life span has not been spent, we have a right to claim God's gift of health AND healing**. And even if that span be past—if it be His will that we should continue here for a time longer—it's equally his will that we should do so in good health. Of course, I mean all who are properly taught and who meet the conditions prescribed in the Word.

You may hear someone say, *"Well, if healing is for all, then we shall never die."* Why not? Divine healing goes no further than the promise of God. God does not promise that we shall never die, but He says:

> *"And you shall serve the LORD your God, and he shall bless your bread, and your water; and I will take sickness away from the midst of you . . . the number of your days I will fulfil."* (Torah: Exodus 23:25-26)

> *"The days of our years are threescore years and ten; and if by reason of strength they be fourscore years . . ."* (Psalm 90:10)

"I said, O my God, take me not away in the midst of my days: your years are throughout all generations." (Psalm 102:24)

"Be not over much wicked, neither be you foolish: why should you die before thy time?" (Ecclesiastes 7:17)

A person might ask, *"Well, how is a person going to die?"* Psalm 104:29 tells us:

"You hide your face, they are troubled: you take away their breath, they die, and return to their dust."

God has given man a certain span of life, and His will is that life should be lived out.

~ CHAPTER TEN ~

HEALING WHEN YOU
LEAST FEEL LIKE IT

Discouragement can rob you of healing and of success in any endeavor—if you let it. When King David was discouraged—his men were ready to stone him—he encouraged himself in the LORD. **Stand up on the inside** and let the Holy One of Israel heal you by His Son: Messiah Jesus.

Discouragement is like a blanket of death. **It can paralyze you with inaction, loss of faith, and no hope**. Discouragement is a tool of the devil. The enemy of your soul wants you to STOP ACTION: he wants you to stop believing for MIRACLES, and for the touch of God in your life.

Let's look for a moment at the definitions of "discouragement."

1. Preventing something from happening by making it more difficult or unpleasant.

2. Trying to stop a person from doing something.

3. Making somebody feel less motivated, confident, or optimistic.

The 15th Century root from the Old French word "descoragier" means "to deprive of courage."

Discouragement can rob you of healing and of success in any endeavor **if you let i**t.

Satan, the devil, is a REAL spirit being. He does NOT want you to succeed in anything. The only success he wants you to have is for his purposes. And, your soul—including the destruction of your mental and physical well being—is his purpose. That's what he is after. The enemy wants your soul: for eternity, and, my friend, **PART of eternity is NOW**.

When Messiah was on earth, He told us: *"The thief (the devil) comes not, but for to steal, and to kill, and to destroy: I am come that they might have life, and that they might have it more abundantly."* (Brit Chadashah / Yochanan [John] 10:10)

It is the devil's will—and goal—to destroy your health, your wealth, and your joy. *"The JOY of the LORD is your strength."* (Tanakh / Ketuvim: Nehemiah 8:10) The Good News is that, **it is the WILL of the LORD**, Jesus the Messiah, **for you to have life more abundantly**. This includes your health, your wealth, and your joy.

Whether you are healthy and successful—or sick and in poverty—the devil's goal is the same. As a matter of fact, the enemy loves to kick people when they are down. He is a major bully.

This is WHY you have to take a stand: first of all spiritually, then mentally and physically.

When King David's followers were thinking about stoning him, after their loss at Ziklag (1 Samuel 30:6) the Bible tells us, *"David encouraged himself in the LORD his God."*

When you are discouraged, you have to STAND UP on the inside and encourage yourself in the LORD. You must remind yourself:

▪ God is for you.

- God loves you and sent His Son, Yeshua (Jesus) the Messiah, as your Atonement.

- God has provided healing—spiritual, mental, and physical—in that atonement. *"With His stripes we are healed."* (Tanakh: Isaiah Chapter 53)

Trust Messiah today ... call upon Him NOW! **Ask Him to save you and heal you.** Pray this prayer:

"God of Abraham, Isaac, and Jacob, I WAS discouraged but NOW I am going to stand up on the inside and resist the devil. I ask you to reveal to me if Yeshua (Jesus) is really my Messiah. Please save me and heal me. Thank you!"

Isaiah Chapter 53 in the Tanakh is a wonderful **prophecy 750 years before time about Messiah's sacrifice for you to purchase your healing.** Read it below:

"Who hath believed our message? And to whom has the arm of JHWH [the LORD] been revealed?

For he grew up before him as a tender plant, and as a root out of a dry ground: he has no form nor comeliness;

and when we see him, there is no beauty that we should desire him.

He was despised, and rejected of men; a man of sorrows, and acquainted with grief: and as one from whom men hide their face he was despised; and we esteemed him not.

Surely he hath borne our griefs, and carried our sorrows; yet we did esteem him stricken, smitten of God, and afflicted.

*But he was wounded for our transgressions, he was bruised for our iniquities; the chastisement of our peace was upon him; and **with his stripes we are healed**.*

All we like sheep have gone astray; we have turned everyone to his own way; and YHWH hath laid on him the iniquity of us all.

He was oppressed, yet when he was afflicted he opened not his mouth; as a lamb that is led to the slaughter, and as a sheep that before its shearers is dumb, so he opened not his mouth.

By oppression and judgment he was taken away; and as for his generation, who [among them] considered that he was cut off out of the land of the living for the transgression of my people to whom the stroke (was due)?

And they made his grave with the wicked, and with a rich man in his death; although he had done no violence, neither was any deceit in his mouth.

Yet it pleased JHWH to bruise him; he hath put him to grief: when thou shall make his soul an offering for sin, he shall see [his] seed, he shall prolong his days, and the pleasure of JHWH shall prosper in his hand.

He shall see of the travail of his soul, [and] shall be satisfied: by the knowledge of himself shall my righteous servant justify many; and he shall bear their iniquities.

Therefore will I divide him a portion with the great, and he shall divide the spoil with the strong; because he poured out his soul unto death, and was numbered with the transgressors: yet he bare the sin of many, and made intercession for the transgressors."

- Isaiah Chapter 53 (Tanakh)

~ CHAPTER ELEVEN ~
HOW TO BE HEALED
BY THE WORD OF GOD

Physical and mental healing belong to you as much as spiritual healing. In this chapter, you will learn HOW to obtain **your healing** from the Word of God. You will find examples AND promises from God for your healing!

Yeshua fulfilled what Isaiah the prophet said 750 years before in Isaiah Chapter 53:4-5.

- He bore **our** sicknesses and diseases.

- He carried away **our** pains.

- With his stripes **WE ARE HEALED.**

Yeshua's body and mind took punishment for **us** ... his blood paid for **our** sins. His body was beaten, wounded, and bruised (even before he was crucified) and then he was nailed to the wooden cross ... FOR **OUR** HEALING: spiritual, physical, and mental!

Oppression—both mental and physical—are included in Yeshua's work for **us**. Messiah was driven; he was abased and looked down upon. Isaiah 53:7 says, **"He was oppressed and he was afflicted ..."** In Isaiah 53:4, where it reads, **" ... he carried our 'pains' ..."**, the literal Hebrew meaning is **"acute pain; intense suffering: MENTAL or PHYSICAL."** What Yeshua did FOR you, you don't have to do!

Yeshua healed the separation between God and man through his work FOR US, and therefore ended Satan's dominion over ALL who would trust in Messiah! *"For this purpose the Son of God was manifested, that he might destroy the works of the devil."* (1 John 3:8)

Yeshua **"carried"** sickness, sin, disease, poverty, and oppression—the works of the devil (Satan)—FOR YOU. Now you don't have to carry them any longer. They do NOT belong to the believer in Messiah Yeshua!

WHAT JESUS DID FOR YOU
YOU DON'T HAVE TO DO!

Now that you know that physical and mental healing belong to the believer in Christ—as much as

spiritual healing—you need to know HOW to obtain it: HOW TO BE HEALED!

One of the avenues through which to obtain—and to minister—Messiah's healing power is by the Word of God.

The Holy Bible says, *"He sent his word, and healed them, and delivered them from their destructions."* (Psalm 107:20.) God's Word heals: **God's nature is healing, and He has given LIFE to his Word**. You can be healed by knowing what God promises in his Word concerning healing. Find the promises God has made you in the Holy Bible for healing and for health, and then appropriate one or more of these promises for yourself.

Speak the promises of God to yourself (or to others). Your faith will rise as you do. *"So then faith comes by hearing, and hearing by the Word of God."* (Romans 10:17) As you confess (or speak aloud) the promises of God, your healing will come. Don't worry if you don't see your healing as soon as you think you should ... it has to happen!

Messiah Jesus taught that what you speak will come to pass if you believe it in your heart (Mark 11:23). Don't talk sickness, or doubt, or unbelief anymore—start talking healing, faith, and belief—based upon what your Father God has promised you! Hearing and meditating upon the Word of God produce healing, also.

I have known people to be healed of conditions they have had for years by **hearing** God's Word while I was preaching (both in worship services indoors and preaching outdoors).

"And they went forth, and preached everywhere, the Lord working with them, and confirming the word with signs following." (Mark 16:20)

Meditating (thinking deeply or fixing attention) upon God's Word brings life and health, also. Proverbs 4:20-22 tells us:

"My son, attend to my words; incline [or, direct] your ear unto my sayings. Let them not depart from your eyes; keep them in the middle of your heart. For they are LIFE unto those that find them, and HEALTH to all their flesh."

~ CHAPTER TWELVE ~
HEALING FROM A
STRANGER IN YOUR BODY

Beverly Mitchell of Douglasville, Georgia (USA), returned home after a vacation to Greece. Much to her surprise she discovered that her house was NOT as she had left it. When she entered the house she could see that someone was redecorating. Carpet torn out, rooms repainted, photos on the walls of people she did NOT know. Washing machine and dryer installed that she did NOT own. A dog she did NOT own. A woman wearing her clothes she did NOT know. And the electrical utilities had been changed to the name of another person.

This is a strange thing to happen. **Another person** you do NOT know taking over your house. However, this is WHY many people are sick physically as well as mentally. **Another being** has take over their house: taken over their body or mind. That other being is a spirit of affliction: **a demon spirit sent by Satan to oppress with the end result of illness, disease, or breakdown.**

Remember, Yeshua taught, *"The thief (Satan) only comes to steal, kill, and destroy."* But the Good News is, *"(Yeshua) came that you may have life, and that you may have it abundantly."* (John 10:10)

SOME PEOPLE ARE BOUND BY A DEMON SPIRIT OF INFIRMITY

There was a woman who had a spirit of infirmity 18 years, and she was bent over, and could not in any way straighten herself up. When Yeshua saw her, he called her, and said to her, **"Woman, you are freed from your infirmity."** He laid his hands on her, and immediately she stood up straight, and glorified God. (Luke 13:11-13 – See also Mark 9:25 and Matthew 8:16)

YOU CAN CAST OUT THE DEMON SPIRITS WITH THE NAME OF YESHUA (JESUS)

*"These signs will accompany those who believe: **in my name** they will cast out demons."* (Mark 16:17)

SPEAK TO THE DEMON SPIRITS AND COMMAND THEM TO LEAVE

The seventy returned with joy, *"Lord, even the demons are subject to us **in your name!**"* (Luke 10:17)

FIRST, BIND SATAN IN THE NAME OF JESUS, AND THEN CAST OUT THE DEMONS

Yeshua said, *"If I by the Spirit of God (Ruach Elohim) cast out demons, then the Kingdom of God has come upon you. How can one enter into the house of the strong man, and plunder his goods, unless he **first bind the strong man**? Then he will plunder his house."* (Matthew 12:28-29)

*"If Satan has risen up against himself, and is divided, he cannot stand, but has an end. But no one can enter into the house of the strong man to plunder, unless he **first binds the strong man**; and then he will plunder his house."* (Mark 3:26-27)

ASK JESUS TO BE YOUR LORD – THEN USE HIS NAME TO CAST OUT DEMONS

Jesus taught, *"Whatever things you will bind on earth will be bound in heaven, and whatever things you will loose on earth will be loosed in heaven."* (Matthew 18:18)

YOU DO NOT HAVE TO TAKE SICKNESS OR DISEASE OR PAIN

When evening came, they brought to Yeshua many people who were possessed with demons. **He cast out the spirits with a word, and healed all who were sick**, so that it might be fulfilled which was spoken through Isaiah the prophet, saying: *"He took our infirmities, and bore our diseases."* (Matthew 8:16-17)

THE NAME YESHUA (JESUS) IS ABOVE THE NAMES SICKNESS, DISEASE, AND PAIN.

USE JESUS' NAME IN FAITH AND CAST OUT THE STRANGERS IN THE HOUSE.

"Therefore God also highly exalted him, and gave to him the Name which is above every name; that at the name of Yeshua (Jesus) every knee should bow, of those in heaven, those on earth, and those under the earth, and that every tongue should confess that Yeshua (Jesus) is LORD, to the glory of God the Father." (Philippians 2:9)

~ CHAPTER THIRTEEN ~
THE PROMISES AND THE
PROVISION FOR HEALING

It is God's will for you to be healed in every area of your life; and to maintain that healing: to walk in health! **The most important thing to know is that you do not have to be sick.** Yeshua (Jesus) came to earth to heal. He took your sicknesses, your pains, your diseases—and your sins—on him, and with his stripes **you are healed**.

Jesus' body and mind took the punishment for your sins ... his sinless blood paid the price to buy you back to God. **What Adam lost by disobedience, Jesus won back through obedience**. Spiritual death, which resulted in physical death—*as well as sickness and disease*—was healed. The separation between man and God was ended for all who BELIEVE.

Now ... you can be healed. You have the **PROMISES** in God's Word ... and you have the **PROVISION** Jesus made for you in His atonement: the

finished work obtained by His **onetime—FINAL—supreme sacrifice** for your wholeness. If you want to meet the Healer, Jesus the Anointed One, *NOW* is the time! **Invite God's Son to come into your life by praying this prayer**:

> *"Lord Jesus, I know that you are The Great Physician. You loved me enough to shed your sinless blood and die for me on the cross stake that I might be healed. I know you are alive. Please forgive my sins, come into my life, and be my Master. Help me to live for you, and take me to Heaven when I die."*

If you prayed that prayer and meant it, then you have eternal life and your sins are ALL forgiven. You have been healed in your spirit. Know that God has heard and answered your prayer! The Bible says, *"Whoever shall call upon the name of the LORD shall be saved."* (Romans 10:13) Notice, God did NOT say *"may be saved"*—*"might be saved"*—or even *"probably,"* but his promise is: ***"Whoever shall call … SHALL BE saved!"***

If you need physical or mental healing, pray and ask the Jesus, the Son of God, to heal you … NOW! Or, obtain healing through any of the other methods God has made available:

- The Word of God

- Laying On of Hands

- Passover and the Holy Communion

- Anointing with Oil

- Prayer and Proper Mental Attitude

Know that healing is yours because of:

- The **PROMISES** of God in his Word; and,

- The **PROVISION** of Messiah in His Work for you!

Now that you know YOUR RIGHT to divine healing and health, God wants you to share this Good News with others so they can be healed. **Many times people find healing as they are helping others to be healed.** It is a spiritual law that *"what a man sows, that he also reaps."*

As you lead others to the knowledge of healing and health through Messiah Jesus, you will be "sowing" for your own harvest of divine healing and health.

"Freely you have received, freely give."

~ CHAPTER FOURTEEN ~
HEALING FROM
BIPOLAR DISORDER

While studying Economics, I memorized the following from a book I was reading (I also gave this while delivering my victory and acceptance message during my senior year when voted unanimously by all fraternities—and the independents on campus—for being the "Most Worthless Senior.")

Our system is depressive manic;

It runs from boom and then to panic.

In view of this it would be wise,

for government to stabilize.

And that knowing the need for both

stability and economic growth,

(the economy) can often be a disappointment,

even during constant, steady, full employment!

72

I'm not sure, but I think that was from a book by J. Sullivan Edwards, titled: *Ride the Wild Horses.*

Editor's Note: Even though I won the award for being the "Most Worthless Senior," four years later—while alone in a room—the Mashiach of Israel made me worthy!!! I read a scripture from the Prophet Isaiah in the Tanakh that said; *"Come now, and let us reason together, says the LORD: though your sins be as scarlet, they shall be as white as snow; though they be red like crimson, they shall be as wool."* (Isaiah 1:18) I stood on my bed and lifted my hand to Heaven and said, *"Yeshua, I know you're there, take my hand."* I've never been the same since.

Anyway ... back to *"Our system is depressive manic ..."* Bipolar disorder is a condition where people alternate between periods of a very good or irritable mood and depression. The "mood swings" between mania and depression may be sudden. Not realized by many people, bipolar disorder begins manifesting between the ages of 15 to 25 and seems to have a genetic relationship, whether inherited or transferred by association.

Let me share some statistics about bipolar disorder (BD):

- BD is the fifth leading cause of disability in the world;

- BD is the ninth leading cause of years lost to death or disability in the world;

- BD victims have a suicide rate 60 times higher than the general population;

- BD victims are at higher risk of substance abuse or other mental problems;

- BD usually happens to males earlier in life than females.

Mood swings can alternate from the lows of depression to the highs of mania. During depression a person may feel sad, lose hope, and lose interest in activities that normally give them pleasure. **Mood shifts may happen a few times a year or several times a day**. And, on occasion, mood shifts may happen simultaneously. Most victims of bipolar disorder are treated with medication and / or psychotherapy (psychological counseling). It is the purpose of my teaching here to present you with an alternate method of healing ... and one which may be not only instantaneous, but permanent.

First, let me state that **lots of people suffering from BD do NOT know they have it, or that they need help**. Of those who do know they suffer from the condition, some do NOT want help, especially while they are in a phase of mania. I am assuming that if someone referred you to book chapter, that YOU need help ... or know someone who does.

Bipolar disorder can be caused by any of the following, or a combination thereof:

- Poor nutrition;

- Substance abuse;

- Genetic pre-conditions;

- Associative or learned behavior from a close relative;

- Life changes (like childbirth or death of a loved one);

- Periods of sleeplessness;

- Separation from loved ones;

- Demonic oppression.

NOTE: See "**Addendum**" for manifestations that appear similar to Bipolar Disorder but are the result of different cause.

Let's start with this premise: Nothing is too hard for the LORD. The word of the LORD came to Jeremiah, the Prophet, saying: *"Behold, I am the LORD, the God of all flesh: is there any thing too hard for me?"* (Tanakh: Jeremiah 32:27)

In this chapter **I am going to teach you HOW to pray for the healing of someone who suffers from bipolar disorder**. If YOU are the victim of BD, then just follow the steps and apply them to yourself. Keep in mind, that normally, the person involved **must WANT** healing; however, it is—at times—possible to bring complete healing to a person who does NOT want it, and they can be FREE from the affliction. This is usually the case where demon oppression, or possession, is involved. It is **no more difficult** of a case for the LORD than any other type of demonic activity.

Follow these steps:

Tell the person that God loves them. Explain to the person how Yeshua (Jesus) paid not only for their sins, but also their sickness, disease, pain, and disorders when He shed His life's BLOOD on the cross-stake. (You may want to read Isaiah Chapter 53, verses 4-6 and Matthew Chapter 8, verses 16-17 to them.)

Lead the person in a prayer of wholeness. Have them pray this prayer: *"God in Heaven, I ask you to forgive my sins and to wash me clean in the BLOOD that your Son, Messiah Jesus, shed for me on the cross-stake. I ask Jesus to take control of my life—to be my Lord —and to HEAL me."*

NOTE: If this is a serious case of demonic activity, then lay your hands on them and bind Satan and his hosts in the name of Jesus (Yeshua). Cast the demons out and command Satan and his demons to "cease and desist" their activity in this person: to leave and never come back. Pray a prayer like this:

"Satan, in the name of Jesus I bind you and your spirits who are afflicting this person and command you to stop this affliction, and to leave and never come back. I break your hold on them in the name of the LORD and speak Messiah's BLOOD against you and over this person."

Give the person a Bible and tell them to read in the New Testament starting with the Gospel of John. Follow up with them three (3) times a day—or whatever is convenient—by phone and / or email and give them healing scriptures. (See the Bonus section at the end of this book.) Also, review Chapter Two again.

Take them to Synagogue or Church and to small group Bible studies.

Then ... teach them HOW to pray for others!

Before you leave them, tell them that IF they want "SUPER HIGHS" along with POWER to serve the LORD, to **ask God to baptize them in the the Holy Spirit.** You may want to pray for them right there and lead them into the Holy Spirit Baptism. Study the book, *How to Receive God's Power with Gifts of the Holy Spirit.*

ADDENDUM

I did NOT cover this previously in this chapter, but lots of people who truly know the LORD have similar manifestations of Bipolar Disorder. In the cases I have counseled this has usually been traced to **one of two sources that caused the condition.**

ERROR #1 - The person made a KEY decision based upon inaccurate input. That is, the felt what they were considering was the will of God for them. They had missed God—usually—because they were NOT reading His Word, the Holy Bible, and seeking to know His will. In other cases they were unduly influenced by other people ... or, forces.

Or ...

ERROR #2 - They made a bad decision and even though they later did NOT have peace about it, **"stuck" with that decision** because they did NOT want to be "double minded" (an unstable person) according to the scripture in James Chapter One, verses 5-8.

THE ANSWER: If you are walking with the LORD in daily prayer and Bible study, follow your heart. What is your human spirit (the inner man, the heart) saying to you as the Holy Spirit leads you?

God richly bless you on your journey of wellness!

~ CHAPTER FIFTEEN ~
THE LORD IS YOUR PHYSICIAN

In the 39th year of King Asa's rule, he was diseased in his feet until his disease was very critical. Yet, in his disease, he did not seek the Lord, but went to the physicians for help. He died two years later. You can read about that in 2 Chronicles 16:11-13.

There is nothing wrong with going to physicians or seeking medical help or advice. **But what we should do is seek the Lord first to see what he wants us to do**. He may want to heal us by His sovereign power, over a period of time, or instantaneously.

What you must know:

■ You must know that healing belongs to you.

■ There is no need for you to depart from health.

■ You can be healed ... walk in health ... and help others to do the same.

The dictionary defines "**disease**" as: 1) **Any departure from a state of health**; 2) **A disordered condition of mind or body marked by definite symptoms**.

To be at "ease" is to be FREE from pain or any discomfort, including anxiety and stress. "Dis-ease" is the opposite. **In the Holy Bible, God promised MORE than healing for his people.** He promised DIVINE HEALTH: freedom from disease!

"If you will carefully listen to the voice of the Lord your G-d, and will do that which is right in his sight, and will give ear to his commandments, and keep all his statutes, I will put none of these diseases upon you ... for I am the LORD that heals you." (TORAH: Exodus 15:26)

Notice the last phrase: *"I am the LORD that heals you."* The Hebrew passage is saying, "**I am Jehovah Rapha.**" The Hebrew word "**rapha**" means "**cure, heal, physician, make whole.**" Literally, this passage is saying, "**I am YHWH your physician.**" It is wonderful to be able to claim God's promises for divine healing, but it is even better to walk in **divine HEALTH**: not needing to be healed!

Exodus 23:25 says, *"And you shall serve the LORD your God and he shall bless your bread, and your water; and I will take sickness away from the midst of you."* When sickness is "away" from you, then you have HEALTH. **Thank God, it is His will for YOU to walk in divine health just as much as it is for your soul to be saved.** In 3 John (Yochanan), verse 2, (of the Brit Chadasha)—a passage of scripture which is written to Hebrew Christians and Gentile Christians—the Holy Bible says:

"Beloved, I wish above all things that you may prosper and be in health, even as your soul prospers."

~ CHAPTER SIXTEEN ~
HEALING BY DISCERNING MESSIAH:
A LESSON FROM TORAH

Many people can recite from memory John 3:16, which tells us:

"For God so loved the world that He gave His only begotten Son, that whoever believes in Him should not perish but have everlasting life."

Yeshua said this after mentioning the Torah account of Numbers Chapter 21 which tells us:

"And the people journeyed from mount Hor by the way of the Red sea, to compass the land of Edom: and the soul of the people was much discouraged because of the way.

And the people spoke against God, and against Moses, Wherefore have you brought us up out of Egypt to die in the wilderness? For there is no bread, neither is there any water; and our soul loathes this light bread.

And the LORD sent fiery serpents among the people, and they bit the people; and much people of Israel died.

Therefore, the people came to Moses, and said, We have sinned, for we have spoken against the LORD, and against you; pray unto the LORD, that he take away the serpents from us. And Moses prayed for the people.

And the LORD said unto Moses, Make you a fiery serpent, and set it upon a pole: and it shall come to pass, that every one that is bitten, when he looks upon it, shall live.

And Moses made a serpent of brass, and put it upon a pole, and it came to pass, that if a serpent had bitten any man, when he beheld the serpent of brass, he lived."

The Torah contains many examples ... or types ... of the Messiah to come. It is beautiful that when Messiah was here on earth He quoted from this passage concerning Himself, as He did on many other occasions.

Moshe (Moses) proclaimed, *"Everyone that is bitten (by the serpents), when he looks upon it (the serpent of brass upon the pole) shall live."*

Can you imagine a person almost dead, laying in the desert sand, straining to look at the serpent on the pole ... or a mother with a child almost dead, pointing her child to look at the brass serpent upon the pole.

No one questioned whether they would be healed. For they were told by Moses, *"Whoever looks will be healed."* They knew "whoever" meant them!

As Moses lifted up the serpent in the wilderness, and whoever looked upon it lived, so Messiah would be lifted up on the cross stake, and **whoever believes in Him,** *"should not perish, but have eternal life."*

And so it is that **whoever discerns the Messiah Yeshua lifted up upon the cross stake will be healed: spiritually, mentally, and physically**.

You might wonder how the sinless Messiah would be represented by the example, or type, of a venomous snake. In the Brit Chadashah, 2 Corinthians 5:21 tells us: *"For he hath made Him to be sin for us, who knew no sin; that we might be made the righteousness of God in Him."* This was a fulfillment of Isaiah's prophecy in the Tanakh, *"And the LORD has laid on him the iniquity of us all."* (Isaiah 53:6)

Messiah, on the cross stake, became sin for us by taking our sins upon Himself; and therefore became cursed as the serpent was cursed, that **those who are under the curse might be redeemed from it.**

Sin and sickness are a double curse, and so **the atonement by Messiah is a double cure!** As people who were bitten looked up to the brazen serpent on the pole were healed ... so **those today who are sick and diseased and in pain look upon Messiah, who was lifted up upon the cross stake, are healed.**

The atonement described in the Tanakh in Isaiah Chapter 53 was fulfilled by Messiah Yeshua 750 years later. We are told in Mattiyahu (Matthew) 8:16-17:

"When the even was come, they brought unto Him many that were possessed with devils: and He cast out the spirits with his word, and healed all that were sick: That it might be fulfilled which was spoken by Esaias the prophet, saying, Himself took our infirmities, and bare our sicknesses."

By His stripes you are healed!

~ CHAPTER SEVENTEEN ~
HEALING BY ATTENDING
TO THE WORD OF GOD

In the Proverbs we are instructed as follows:

*"My son, **attend** to my words. Turn your **ear** to my sayings. Let them not depart from your **eyes**. Keep them in the midst of your **heart**. For they are **life** to those who find them, And **health** to their whole body."* (Proverbs 4:20-22)

To **attend** means: **to be present, to focus, to think about**.

This passage shows us **HOW to attend to the Words of God**: His PROMISES of healing.

- ▌ We must have an **attentive ear**.

- ▌ We must have a **steady and fixed look**.

- ▌ We must have an **receptive heart**.

There are so many promises in the word of God that pertain to divine healing and health. We have covered many of them in previous chapters. However, if you are in need of healing NOW, it is very helpful—and in some cases, extremely important—to attend to these promises by:

- An **attentive ear**;

- A **steady and fixed look**; and,

- A **receptive heart**.

Listen to the promises. If you do not have access to some means of hearing via a recorded message, then just **speak the promises aloud to yourself**. I do this every day. I have been on Planet Earth a long time. I was just to my doctor for my annual physical last week and at the end—and, after looking over laboratory tests—he asked me, *"Do you want to come back in one or two years?"*

It is good to feel healthy. And, **health** is not only a **gift** from God, but a **promise** from God.

Look at the promises. Read them and look closely at them. **Focus on them** by meditating upon them: through your eyes AND in your mind. This way you will be able to **SEE** them at any time on the screen of your mind (if not verbatim, at least the content of the promises). They are your life blood—literally—when you need healing. That is **WHY** God has given them to you.

Receive the promises. Think about the **gift** which God is offering you. **A gift has to be received.** Realize that God loves you so much that He has provided healing for you through His Son: Yeshua Ha Mashiach (Jesus the Messiah). Healing—and, divine health—are yours through the **provision** of Messiah by His atonement on the cross stake (*"And with his stripes we are healed."),* and the **promises** of God in His Word.

Life and **health** are yours according to the promise of God in Proverbs 4:20-22.

If you have read my teachings on healing and health you know that I am NOT against doctors or seeking medical help. However, make sure God wants you to go to the doctor or to seek medical help. Pray first, and ask God what he wants you to do. He may want to heal you instantly (or, over a period of time) without medical help. Study my book, *Health and Healing Complete Guide to Wholeness.*

The question is: *"Whose word will you take?"* The word of a doctor, a friend ... or the Word of God. God does NOT lie, and He promises **healing** and **health** to you if you fulfill the conditions.

~ CHAPTER EIGHTEEN ~
HEALING FROM ANGER

Anger can result in depression, anxiety, or other illnesses. And, it can work itself out in motivating pornography use, divorce, and even church, synagogue, or workplace dissension. At the least, anger can cause us to say something or do something that might hurt another individual or group of people.

Unforgiveness, if not dealt with, can produce anger. However, lots of things can cause anger. Even seemingly small things like being overlooked in the decision making process (at home, at the office, or in a group setting such as at synagogue or church): Especially when one is **not** consulted in a decision or action relating to them.

Many times a person will do or say subtle little things to irritate someone with whom they are angry.

All of us get angry at times. We are human, and we have a full spectrum of emotions. So, when we are offended, we become angry. However, anger that is NOT resolved, just like any other emotional problem, can result in **serious** illness: spiritual, physical, and mental.

The Holy Bible tells us, *"Be angry and do not sin; do not let the sun go down upon your wrath; neither give place to the devil."* This scriptural admonition shows that anger is a part of the human psyche, but that it must be dealt with, and that stated: **no longer than by the end of the day**. My father used to tell us, *"Don't go to bed mad."*

When we do NOT deal with anger properly, we allow a wall to be built up, and each successive hour or day the wall gets wider and taller and stronger. It actually becomes a **stronghold** of the enemy. And quite probably, this is WHY the situation(s) that caused the anger were designed in the pit of Hell itself, by none other than Satan, the enemy of your soul.

Satan hates you. So he utilizes people and demons to hurt you: spiritually, mentally, or physically. And if he can make you **angry** in the process, he will then have a cycle of destruction established. If you are NOT successful in breaking this cycle, then it will become self propagating. That is WHY you need to **resolve the issue of anger**. Usually, the issue of anger can be resolved in the following ways:

- Forgiving the offender(s);

- Settling differences; and,

- Practicing (or, learning) self-control.

Sometimes it is NOT always possible to settle differences, especially if you have NOT done anything wrong. However, you can always FORGIVE and let God settle the matter. *"Forgiving others, as God, for Messiah's sake has forgiven you."*

If an attempt to settle differences is going to exacerbate, or worsen, the situation, then leave it in God's hands. Place the other party (the offender) into God's hands, *"Avenge not yourselves, but rather* **give place unto wrath***: for it is written, Vengeance is mine; I will repay, says the Lord."*

To **give place unto wrath**, then, is to leave it for God to come in and execute wrath or vengeance on the enemy. **Do not execute wrath yourself. Leave it to God**. Commit all to him. Leave yourself and your enemy in his hands, assured that he will vindicate you and punish your enemy. (I have seen this happen many times.)

Never be afraid to confront when you have prayed into the situation, and never **lose** your temper (or, your anger). *"Let every one be quick to listen, slow to speak, and slow to get angry; For the anger of man does not forward the righteous purpose of God."* **Maintain self control**. *"For God hath not given us the spirit of fear; but of power, and of love, and of a sound mind (or, self-control)."* – 2 Timothy 1:7

Remember: the devil, Satan, hates you, but **Messiah, Jesus, loves you**. The Bible says, *"The thief (the devil) comes to steal, to kill, and to destroy. But Jesus (the Good Shepherd) comes that you might have LIFE, and have it abundantly."*

~ CHAPTER NINETEEN ~
HEALING MIRACLES
BY THE MERCY OF GOD

It is an eternal truth that the LORD never changes.

"For I, YHWH, do not change; therefore you, sons of Jacob, are not consumed." (Tanakh: Malachi 3:6)

"Yeshua Ha Mashiach is the same yesterday, today, and forever." (Brit Chadashah: Hebrews 13:8)

The nature of God never changes. One of the covenant names of Ha Shem is **YHWH RAPHA**, which in Hebrew means **"The LORD our Physician," or "The LORD our Healer."**

"If you will diligently listen to the voice of YHWH your God, and will do that which is right in his eyes, and will pay attention to his commandments, and keep all his statutes, I will put none of the diseases on you, which I have put on the Egyptians; for I am YHWH who heals you." (Torah: Exodus 15:26)

95

Rapha is a primitive root in the Hebrew language and means **"mend, cure, heal, physician, repair, make whole."**

The mercy of the LORD endures forever. *"O give thanks unto the LORD; for he is good; for his mercy endures forever."* (2 Chronicles 16:34)

Even nature reveals the attitude of God toward the healing of our bodies. As soon as disease enters your body, the natural immune system begins to attack. If sickness were the will of God, then the Creator would NOT have designed your body with the marvelous systemic attack on disease and the ability of your auto immune system to fight and ward off disease.

If sickness, disease, and pain were the will of God, then it would be sin to go to the doctor, or to use medicine, or to attempt to delete malevolent works in your spirit, mind, or body. As an extension of this model of thought (which is prevalent in much of Judaism as well as Christianity), it would be SIN to pray to God for alleviation from your sickness, disease, or pain.

It would be SIN to pray for God to heal you if it were the will of God for you to have sickness, disease, or pain.

But NO, thank the LORD **it is his will for us to be healed** and to walk in health. That it his nature: healing. He is YHWH your physician. And his nature never changes.

The attitude of Messiah Yeshua toward healing while he was on earth is shown by the fact that he was **everywhere** moved with compassion.

*A great multitude of people "came to hear him, and to be healed of their diseases; and they that were vexed with unclean spirits (demons): **and they were healed**. And the whole multitude sought to touch him: for there went virtue (power) out of him, and **healed them all**."* (Brit Chadashah: Luke 6:17-19).

*"Now when the sun was setting, all they that had any sick people with different diseases brought them unto him; and **he laid his hands on every one of them, and healed them**. And demons also came out of many, crying out, and saying, 'You are Messiah the Son of God. And he, rebuking them, allowed them not to speak: for they (the demons) knew that he was Messiah."* (Brit Chadashah: Luke 4:40-41)

Messiah said, *"If you have seen me, you have seen the Father."* The healing nature of God was manifested in the life and ministry of Yeshua. God has never withdrawn his healing compassion. Yeshua has never withdrawn his healing compassion. The nature of God is eternal. He is your doctor: your healer.

If you believe in God, then you believe He exists. And, if He exists, then He can still heal you.

- He wants to heal you.

- He promised to heal you.

- He will heal you.

"Praise the LORD, my soul, and forget not all his benefits;

***Who forgives all your sins; Who heals all your diseases**;*

Who redeems your life from destruction; Who crowns you with lovingkindness and tender mercies;

Who satisfies your desire with good things, So that your youth is renewed like the eagle's." – Psalm 103:2-5

~ CHAPTER TWENTY ~
HEALING FOR BODY
AND MIND ABUSE

Physical and mental abuse can hinder healing. The psychosomatic forces that block healing are very strong: however, in opposition to much modern writing on this subject – psycho physiological problems can be healed instantly. I have seen multitudes of people healed through the laying on of hands, and many times through praise alone.

Many disorders have their source in the stress and strain of everyday activity or concern. For example, high blood pressure and lower back pain. There are, however, more complex inter-related issues that evolve from physical and mental abuse, even of pre-natal history. **Abuse in the womb—physical or mental—is an area that requires the Gift of the Word of Knowledge and / or the Word of Wisdom, accompanied with prayer for healing**. And, sometimes the Gift of Discernment accompanied by deliverance.

Mind-body emotional disorders are covered by Messiah's atonement on the cross-stake.

Yeshua's body and mind took punishment for **us** ... his blood paid for **our** sins. His body was beaten, wounded, and bruised (even before he was crucified) and then he was nailed to the wooden cross ... FOR **OUR** HEALING: spiritual, physical, and mental!

Oppression—both mental and physical—is included in Yeshua's work for **us**. Messiah was driven; he was abased and looked down upon. Isaiah 53:7 says, *"He was oppressed and he was afflicted."* In Isaiah 53:4, where it reads, *"He carried our 'pains'"*, the literal Hebrew meaning is **"acute pain; intense suffering: MENTAL or PHYSICAL."** What Yeshua did FOR you, you don't have to do!

One highly neglected therapeutic healing remedy for physical and mental abuse is the offering of PRAISE to God. The Holy Bible tells us the God lives in the praise of His people. *"But you are holy, O you that inhabits the **praises** of Israel."* (Tanakh: Psalm 22:3)

When you praise God, you are creating an atmosphere for the LORD to invade your situation. I

am convinced, after 45 years of praying for sick and infirm people, that many people have back pain, depression, and other conditions of malevolence in their bodies and their minds because **they do NOT lift their hands and praise God meaningfully**, in sincerity—and often—in frequency.

Praise should be habitual: as much a pattern of life as eating and breathing. Praise can restore you and make your whole outlook on life different. **A positive healing energy from God will saturate your being when you offer praise unto the LORD.** Instead of being downtrodden mentally, which can affect you physically, you will be encouraged. Even problems that are of financial or relational concern can be overcome with praise to God.

Lift your hands NOW. Tell the LORD how much you love Him. Thank Him for sending His Son, Yeshua, to pay for your sins, to heal you, and to deliver you from whatever—or whomever—is troubling you.

Your mind—and therefore your body—can be abused by many things. At times there are hindrances to healing: things or conditions that are causing the sickness or affliction, and that must be dealt with before healing can take place permanently.

Things such as:

- Unforgiveness, bitterness, or resentment (Mark 11:25-26)

- Envy and strife (James 3:16)

- Improper food, rest, sunshine, or exercise (Isaiah 30:15)

- Speaking evil of, or causing harm to, God's ministers (1 Samuel 26:9)

- Involvement in the occult or in witchcraft (Deuteronomy 18:10-12)

- Association with religious cults (1 John 4:1-3 / 1 John 5:20)

Whether sickness is caused by disobeying God through an unforgiving spirit, strife, or resentment, involvement in the occult, or association with religious cults, or even pre-natal abuse, Yeshua Ha Mashiach (the Anointed One) is the answer!

Through PRAYER we can come to God and ask Him to to heal us. We can also ask Him to deliver us, and to forgive us, if necessary! In the Brit Chadashah, 1 Yochanan (John) 1:9 says, *"If we confess our sins, he is faithful and just to forgive us our sins, and to cleanse us from all unrighteousness."* In the Tanakh, Psalm 50:15, we read, *"Call upon me in the day of trouble: I will deliver you, and you shall glorify me."*

Through PRAISE we invite God into our situation. The anointing of the Holy Spirit breaks the yoke of mental and physical oppression. **Lift your hands in PRAISE to God right NOW.**

~ CHAPTER TWENTY-ONE ~
HEALING IS THE HIGHER TRUTH

Healing may be of different types or classifications:

- Instant

- Protracted (over time)

- Miracle

Not all healings may be classified as MIRACLES; however, some **are** miracles; the miracle healings are usually instantaneous.

There is a type of healing that is a MIRACLE but that is NOT specifically a generic healing. For example: restoration of body parts, which will be in evidence more as we approach the last days.

No matter what type of healing you need—spiritual, mental, physical—it is important to realize that you live in a human body that was born of the seed line of Adam: the natural man. **You, therefore, operate under the five sensory perceptions of touch, taste, vision,**

hearing, and smell. Also, there can be a sixth sense of knowing that operates in some people.

I am a pilot, although I have not flown an aircraft for many years. When you are studying for your Commercial and Instrument license(s), you quickly **learn NOT to rely on your sensory perceptions when flying under INSTRUMENT flight rules**.

When you are training, you practice flying with a "hood" on so that you can NOT see outside the airplane; **you can only see the instruments**.

Also, in practice, while inside the classroom you are blindfolded and placed in a revolving chair that spins around. Sometimes you think you are going LEFT when you are going RIGHT. Or, you think you are sitting still when you are spinning. This is because you are depending upon your natural sensory perceptions. However, your inner ear can play tricks on you when your vision is cut off from operation. Vertigo can result from visual irregularities, also.

Many pilots who became scared in limited or no visibility —and **who made a decision to trust their sensory perceptions (their senses) instead of their**

instruments—have died drilling a hole in the ground. I, personally, believe this is how the young John F. Kennedy, Jr. died.

It is the same way with healing. You have to rely on the PROMISES in God's Word. The fact that your body—or, maybe your mind—is sick, is a truth. However, **the PROMISES of healing by God are a HIGHER TRUTH**. As you declare in faith (you must believe) the promise(s) of God for your healing, **the LESSER TRUTH has to come into alignment with the HIGHER TRUTH.**

God will heal you and keep you healthy if you serve Him.

"You will serve the LORD ... and I will take sickness away." (Torah: Exodus 23:25)

God wants to heal you: to save you from disease and sin.

"I am the LORD that heals you." (Torah: Exodus 15:26)

Yeshua, the Messiah, never refused healing to anyone.

"Yeshua went about healing all that were oppressed of the devil." (Acts 10:38)

106

Yeshua's healing nature never changes.

"Yeshua Ha Mashiach is the same yesterday, today, and forever." (Hebrews 13:8)

Make a commitment to the Word of God today. When your body tells you that you are sick, turn to the PROMISES of God. **By Messiah's stripes you are healed.** (Tanakh: Isaiah Chapter 53).

Doctors and medicine can only do so much; but **God can do anything!** Pray, and ask God to show you what to do! *"Behold, I am the LORD, the God of all flesh: is there anything too hard for me?"* (Jeremiah 32:27)

~ CHAPTER TWENTY-TWO ~
HEALING FROM ALIENATION

We receive interesting prayer and email requests from different countries. One of the most common areas of prayer needs among Christians is in the area of "alienation."

To "alienate" means "to cause to feel isolated." It also means **to lose** the **support or sympathy** of a person or people. It can be both proactive and subjective. A person can cause another person or people to feel isolated—or—they can cause themselves to lose the support or sympathy of others by their own actions.

The origin of the of the word "alienate" is from the Latin "alienare" meaning "**estrange**" and the Latin "alius" meaning "**other**." In other words, a person is caused **to feel less close or friendly.**

We should never cause anyone to feel isolated. There is one guideline in Scripture covering a valid reason for separating from another believer (a person who claims to be a Christian), and that is found in 1 Corinthians 5:9-13. The Holy Bible says you should not associate with immoral people. This does NOT mean UNbelievers ... to avoid them you would have to get out of the world completely.

This passage is talking about a person who says they are a brother or sister in the Lord (saved) but who is sexually immoral or greedy, or worships idols, or is a slanderer (gossip) or a drunkard, or lawbreaker. The Apostle Paul says: *"To put away from yourselves the evil person."*

The purpose of this podcast / teaching is not to discuss that kind of alienation. I am talking about the alienation caused by a Christian that is very grievous to the Holy Spirit: **purposely causing another person—Christian or non Christian—to feel isolated, or to cause them to feel they do not have your support or sympathy.**

Follow the example modeled by Messiah Yeshua (Jesus). **He made people feel accepted.** His major confrontations were with the religious crowd, but only because of their religious and hypocritical viewpoints and actions. But even then, He spoke **truth** to them, because He loved them, but never shut them out as individuals.

When Mahatma Ghandi, as a young man, first came to the United States he visited a church; however, they made him sit in the back, evidently because of the color of his skin. Think what a great spiritual force he could have been in the world if he had become a Christian! He admired the teachings of Jesus, but was not himself a Christian.

Che Guevara, the Argentine Marxist activist and revolutionary mass-murderer, as a young boy had a bad experience with a Christian missionary. Think what a great spiritual force he could have been in the world if he had become a Christian!

Both of these men were alienated by Christians. But ... **we** can turn the tide. You and I can believe God to use us to **minister a spirit of acceptance** under the anointing of the Holy Spirit. Pray daily for this.

If physical evil (suffering and death) entered the world through sin (moral evil), then it stands to reason that physical evil can be cured (healed) through righteousness (the opposite of sin). Whenever you feel the urge to alienate a person, stop—back up one step—and **ask the Holy Spirit to come in and anoint you with a spirit of acceptance.**

We will never be at one with ourselves if we are knowingly alienating others! God has made provision for our restoration with Him, with others, and with ourselves!

Alienation from nature is a result of the Fall (of Adam). Alienation from others—also from self and from God—is also a result of the Fall. Messiah Yeshua (Jesus) has purchased our acceptance with His own Blood on the cross-stake. How could we, as His children and representatives, shut out or alienate others! Since God has made it possible for us to be "at one" with Him, we can—if we will to—be at one with others and with ourselves.

Also, **if someone has alienated you, then simply forgive them. God accepts you ... you are His child. You will reap HEALING from alienation by sowing FORGIVENESS.**

~ CHAPTER TWENTY-THREE ~
HOW TO BE SURE
HEALING IS FOR YOU

I want to continue our discussion in this chapter about "Is Healing For Everyone?"

Healing is **still** the will of God as it was in the past. **It is God's will to heal ALL who have need of healing— and to fulfill the number of their days!**

I want you to recall that all those Messiah Yeshua called back from the dead were young people **who had NOT lived out their fullness of years**. And, in that very fact we may see His protest against premature death. **If the allotted span (of life) has not been spent, we have a right to claim God's benefit of promised healing and health**.

And, even though a person's span of 70 to 80 years has been passed, it's equally God's will we should live the extra (extension of years) in good health. If you want to know what's in a person's will (that is, their Last Will and Testament) you have to read the will. People leave a

Last Will and Testament and they write it **before** they die. They don't come back to life and change it AFTER they have died.

Jesus came back to life to minister what He put in His will. **If we want to know God's will on any subject, let us read His will.** For example, let's say someone says, *"My relative who was very wealthy passed away; and, I would like to know if they left me anything in their will."* I will tell them, *"Why don't you read their will and find out."* The word "testament," legally speaking, means a person's will. The Holy Bible contains God's Last Will and Testament: The Old Covenant (Tanakh); and the New Covenant (B'rit Chadashah).

In other words, the New Covenant that Messiah established for His people is what he bequeathed us: all the blessings of redemption, everything purchased by His atonement on the cross stake. His prophesied death and resurrection impacted the glorious ministration of that will. **Since it is Messiah's Last Will and Testament, anything later is a forgery.** Notice I said, "The Last Will and Testament." **It's the New Covenant: He did NOT change it after He was raised from the**

dead. He came to minister the life, healing, and the promises obtained in that New Covenant.

A man never writes a new will after he is dead. If healing is God's will for us, then **to say that the age of miracles is past is virtually saying what is opposite of the truth**: that a will is no good after the death of the testator. **Yeshua is not only the testator who died, He was resurrected and He is also the Mediator of that will, that covenant.**

He is our lawyer, so to speak. Yeshua is our lawyer. He will not beat us out of our rights in the will left to us, as some earthly attorneys do. Messiah Yeshua is our representative at the right hand of our Heavenly Father. And, for the answer to the question under consideration, let us look away from the modern tradition, and go to the Word of God, which is the revelation of His will. In the 15th Chapter of Exodus (in the Torah), just after the passage of God's people through the Red Sea—when the Children of Israel were delivered from cruel Pharaoh and Egypt—an event happened that typified our redemption. And, it was written, as the Holy Bible says, for our admonition.

God gave His first promise to HEAL right after tha event. **This promise was for ALL PEOPLE.** God named the conditions, the conditions were met, and we read, *"He brought them forth also with silver and gold, there was not one feeble person among all their tribes,"* and it is here that God gave the **covenant of healing** revealed by and sealed with His first covenant and His redemptive name: **Jehovah Rapha**, translated **"I am the LORD that heals you,"** OR literally, **"I am Jehovah, your doctor,"** OR **"I am YHWH, your physician."**

This is God's Word, settled in Heaven: a never changing fact concerning God's character; and don't let anyone beat you out of His Will. Don't let anyone—a minister, a rabbi, another person that claims they know the LORD—don't let them tell you that Jesus does NOT do MIRACLES today!

My friend, **Messiah Jesus—Yeshua Ha Mashiach—is the SAME yesterday, today, and forever**. (Hebrews 13:8) And, during His earthly ministry, Yeshua never refused healing to anyone! And, my friend, **He wants to heal you right now**. The POWER of the Ruach Ha

Chodesh (the Holy Spirit) is upon you right now. Receive that MIRACLE you need in the name of Jesus!

~ CHAPTER TWENTY-FOUR ~
HEALING MENTAL DISEASE
AND DEPRESSION

Mental disease and depression may have their root in any of the following, or a combination of them:

- Physical injury;

- Mental injury; or,

- Spiritual injury.

Physical injury may happen due to the following:

- Accidents

- Abuse

- Error in medical diagnosis

- Malnutrition

- Lack of dietary supplements

Mental injury may happen due to the following:

- Accidents

- Abuse

- Prolonged physical stress

- Deferred hope

- Loss of a loved one

- Malnutrition

- Rejection

- Discouragement

- Lack of dietary supplements

- Unattainable or unrealistic goals

- War and chaos

- Genetic provocations

Spiritual injury may happen due to the following:

- Extreme disappointment

- Slander

- Accusations (founded or unfounded)

- Involvement in the occult

- Activity with religious cults

- Loss of a loved one

Also, be aware that **any of the three (3) types of injury mentioned** (physical, mental, or spiritual) **can be a result of demonic activity. It can also be the result of a combination of the demonic and the physical, mental, or spiritual.** For example, a demon spirit may ride in upon (that is, take advantage of) an injury weakness and use it as a channel of possession or oppression.

NOTICE: Physical injury may result in spiritual and mental injury. Spiritual injury may result in physical and mental injury. Mental injury may result in spiritual and physical injury. **They can be inter-related.** This is because **we were created a tripartite being: body, mind, and spirit.**

For example, **a physical injury resulting from an accident can result in mental depression and spiritual regression.** By spiritual regression, I am talking about wandering away from God. A more precise example of this could be bitterness or anger toward God as a result of an accident, or the death of a loved one, or unattainable (unrealistic) goals.

Deferred hope many times is the cause of a person turning away from God; with the possibility of a **twofold prognosis**: **mental injury** (depressive manic and schizophrenic tendencies) and **physical injury** (sickness or disease, and even paralysis).

Somebody reading this message has been hurt. You were crushed in your spirit. You have been depressed and your mind has been confused as a result. The enemy of your soul, Satan, used human enemies (some you did NOT know about) to attack you, malign you, and to attempt to remove you from a place of blessing.

I have GOOD NEWS for you from God. The LORD is going to turn that situation around—promotion and blessing are coming to you unexpectedly—and you will be in a better position to build God's kingdom, and to receive GREAT BLESSING from God for yourself, also.

"We know that all things work together for good to them who love God and are called to His purpose." (Romans 8:28)

"Behold, they shall surely gather together, but not by me: whosoever shall gather together against thee shall fall for your sake." (Isaiah 54:15)

"But I will put it into the hand of them that afflict thee; which have said to your soul, 'Bow down, that we may go over:' and you hast laid your body as the ground, and as the street, to them that went over." (Isaiah 51:23)

Joseph's enemies drove him into the position of Prime Minister where the purposes of God were fulfilled.

Daniel's enemies drove him into the position of Prime Minister where the purposes of God were fulfilled.

Mordecai's enemies drove him into the position of Prime Minister where the purposes of God were fulfilled.

Your enemies can drive **you** into the position of blessing if you will release your faith in Messiah Yeshua, the LAMB of God, Who bought you with the BLOOD of the everlasting Passover.

Love God and live for Him. If you are following His purpose for your life, your enemies will drive you to a better position.

PRAY: Ask God to smite Satan, to turn the situation around which has been designed against you by the enemy, and to use it for your promotion to the glory of God. There will be a performance unto you of the thing spoken to you by the LORD because you believed!

START PRAISING GOD!

I trust this teaching will help you.

~ CHAPTER TWENTY-FIVE ~
ALL HEALING IS POSSIBLE
IF YOU BELIEVE

A man asked Yeshua (Jesus) to pray for his son who was mute and deaf and, also, at times had seizures due to a demon possessing him. Many times from a child the demon had tried to cast him into fire and water to destroy him. (Brit Chadashah: Mark Chapter 9:17-27)

The man asked Yeshua, *"If you can do anything, have compassion on us, and help us."*

Yeshua answered the man, *"If you can?"* *"Believe, all things are possible to him that believes."* (Verse 23)

Immediately the father of the child cried out with tears, *"I believe. Help my unbelief!"*

When Jesus saw that a multitude came running together, he rebuked the unclean spirit, saying to him, *"You mute and deaf spirit, I command you, come out of him, and never enter him again!"*

Having cried out, and convulsed greatly, it (the demon) came out of him. The boy became like one dead; so much that most of them said, *"He is dead."* But Jesus took him by the hand, and raised him up; and he arose."

All healing is possible if you believe. Faith is a gift. Therefore, you can pray and ask the Heavenly Father for faith.

All people have been given faith. The Bible tells us *"to think reasonably, as God has apportioned to each person a measure of faith."* (Romans 12:3) You already have a measure —or, portion—of faith. However, if you want more faith, then ask the LORD to give you more faith like the boy's father in this passage. He cried out to Yeshua, *"I believe. Help my unbelief!"*

Sometimes fasting helps to bring deliverance and healing. However, Jesus does NOT need to fast. He is God. Believe, and if you need more faith, then ask Him to help your unbelief ... to give you more faith. If, however, you feel the Holy Spirit wants you to fast, then do that.

The Holy Spirit, the Ruach Ha Chodesh, is the agent of God on earth to supply the resurrection power of Messiah.

Healing and deliverance have already been purchased for you. **Read Isaiah Chapter 53** in the Tanakh. **The rabbis never read this passage out loud in synagogue because it clearly shows that our sins are forgiven and we are healed by the stripes of the real Passover Lamb of God: Yeshua Ha Mashiach.**

This is the whole point of Passover: it points back to deliverance from the death angel in Egypt, and is an everlasting reminder to have us **apply the BLOOD of the Lamb of God BY FAITH upon the doors of our hearts and home for protection.** For it is by the BLOOD of Messiah that we have deliverance and protection from Satan and his works: sin, sickness, disease, and oppression.

My question to you today is: *"**Can** you believe? **Will** you believe? Do you **want** to believe?"*

If you want to be healed—and if you believe that Jesus can heal you—then all you have to do is believe that **He**

will heal you. Ask Him to heal you NOW. Just tell Him, *"Lord, I believe; help my unbelief."*

The Bible tells us about a woman who came to Messiah Jesus and asked Him to deliver her daughter from a demon who was possessing her.

"Jesus went out from there, and withdrew into the region of Tyre and Sidon.

Behold, a Canaanite woman came out from those borders, and cried, saying, "Have mercy on me, Lord, you son of David! My daughter is severely demonized!"

But he answered her not a word. His disciples came and begged him, saying, "Send her away; for she cries after us."

But he answered, "I wasn't sent to anyone but the lost sheep of the house of Israel."

But she came and worshiped him, saying, "Lord, help me."

*But he answered, "It is not appropriate to take **the children's bread** and throw it to the dogs."*

But she said, "Yes, Lord, but even the dogs eat the crumbs which fall from their masters' table."

Then Yeshua answered her, **"Woman, great is your faith! Be it done to you even as you desire."** *And her daughter was healed from that hour."* (Matthew 15:21-28)

If I put some money in your coat pocket and tell you, *"I put some money in your pocket. I want you to use it for lunch today."* You would probably say *"Thank you,"* and go on your way. Why would you take my word for your lunch money without doubting it, and NOT take the Word of God for your daily bread without doubting it. **Yeshua taught us that healing and deliverance are the children's bread.**

Do NOT quit, my friend. Press in for your healing and deliverance. The LORD is faithful.

~ *CHAPTER TWENTY-SIX* ~
HEALING FROM STRESS

One of the most requested areas of help today is from people suffering from stress.

One medical source defines stress as: *"Forces from the outside world impinging on the individual."* However, I disagree with this definition—or, at least I think it is only a **partial** definition.

As a graduate industrial engineer, I was required to study and know such subject matter as: Strength of Materials, Dynamics, Quantitative and Qualitative Analysis, and, of course, upper level physics and chemistry. I find it interesting that the physical (or, physics) definition of stress is two fold and more correctly applicable to the human genome:

*An applied **external** force or system of forces that tends to strain or deform a body.*

*The **internal** resistance of a body to such an applied force or system of forces.*

Therefore, as pertains to the human condition, we could accurately say that stress (either from external or internal forces) is: *"a mentally, physically, or emotionally disruptive or upsetting condition occurring in response to adverse **external** or **internal** influences and capable of affecting physical health, usually characterized by increased heart rate, a rise in blood pressure, muscular tension, irritability, and depression."*

Since we are a tripartite being (body, mind, spirit) we can reasonably assume that stress can affect us: physically, mentally, and spiritually ... and that, since all three are interconnected, either one may also influence the others. The synergistic effect of which could produce total wreck, or breakdown! This is WHY some people who come to me for help seem to at first be manifesting total meltdown.

Let me give you the four KEY curatives to this, and lesser, conditions:

1. STOP the activities that seem to be causing you stress. If you can not stop them completely, then force yourself to take pre-scheduled breaks for rest or recreation. (A non scheduled break could be as soon as you feel the outset of anxiety or stress.)

2. DO something you enjoy. Find a new hobby or recreation ... do something you have always wanted to do. Ride a motorcycle. Fly an airplane. Build something. Learn to dance.

3. SPEAK affirmations to yourself. Write them on paper, or record them and play them back. The importance is TO SAY them to yourself. The speech mechanism is vitally associated with your central nervous system. You can bring healing and strength to your whole system, especially if you are saying the Word of God. Find scriptures that pertain to: 1. Your situation; and, 2. Your new goals (recreation or desires).

4. PRAY in tongues.

> **A**. When you **pray in tongues**, you are praying according to the will of God, even if you do not understand it. *"He who, when speaking in tongues, **is speaking, not to men, but to God**, for no one understands him; yet **in spirit he is speaking hidden truths**."* (1 Corinthians 14:2)

> **B**. Also, when you even just **sigh (or groan) in tongues**, you are allowing the Holy Spirit to intercede for you according to the will of God, and

thereby bring you therapeutic help. *"Likewise the Spirit also **helps our infirmities: for we know not what we should pray for** as we ought: but **the Spirit itself makes intercession for us** with groanings which cannot be uttered. And **he that searches the hearts knows what is the mind of the Spirit**, because he makes intercession for the saints **according to the will of God.**"* (Romans 8:26-27)

C. One of the great advantages when you **praise God in tongues** is that you are engaged in **pure worship**. There are not enough words in your native language (Hebrew, English, Spanish, etc.) to tell God how wonderful He is, and how much you love Him. However, when you praise Him in tongues, the Holy Spirit (the Ruach HaChodesh) is praising the LORD through you, and God comes on the scene with healing power. The Bible tells us that God lives in the praises of His people. *"But you are holy, You who inhabit the praises of Israel."* (Psalm 22:3)

Lift your hands and PRAISE Him in tongues right now. If you have never received this **POWER,** read the unabridged book by Prince Handley, *How To Receive God's Power with Gifts of the Spirit.*

~ CHAPTER TWENTY-SEVEN ~
HEALING PROMISES ARE FOR FULFILLMENT IN YOUR LIFE

God has given us many promises of healing and health in His Word. We have covered many of these in past podcasts and teachings. However, I want you to notice that **the ONLY PURPOSE of God's promises is their fulfillment in YOUR life**.

God's promises show what He wants to do for us. In the Word of God they are spoken of as "exceeding great and precious" promises. There is NO reason to doubt these promises and we have every reason to EXPECT their fulfillment. Promises such as:

MESSIAH JESUS NEVER REFUSED HEALING TO ANYONE

"Yeshua went about ... healing all that were oppressed of the devil."
[Acts 10:38]

JESUS' HEALING NATURE NEVER CHANGES

133

"Yeshua, the Messiah, the same yesterday, and today, and forever."

[Hebrews 13:8]

GOD PROMISES HEALING AND FORGIVENESS OF SINS TO YOU

"Who forgives all your sins: who heals all your diseases."

[Psalm 103:3]

GOD WANTS TO HEAL

"I am the LORD that heals you."

[Exodus 15:26]

GOD WILL HEAL YOU AND KEEP YOU HEALTHY IF YOU SERVE HIM

"You shall serve the LORD ... and I will take sickness away."

[Exodus 23:25]

ASK THE LORD JESUS TO HEAL YOU NOW ASK HIM TO SAVE YOU

"Call upon me in the day of trouble: I will deliver you."

Yeshua said to the religious crowd of His day: *"My word has NO place in you."* **QUESTION:** Does God's word have a place in **you**? A place of honor, trust, authority … and of faith? If so, then you can BELIEVE what God has promised you and ACT on it by faith.

God is not a man that He should lie, nor the son of man that he should repent. If you are sick, or diseased, or in pain, you have access to the PROMISES of God and the PROVISION of God by the atonement of Messiah Jesus on the cross stake when He took YOUR sins, your sicknesses, your diseases, and your pains UPON HIMSELF for you.

"Surely he has borne our infirmities, and carried our diseases; yet we esteemed him stricken, struck by God, and afflicted. But he was wounded for our transgressions, he was bruised for our iniquities; the chastisement of our peace was on him; and with his stripes we are healed." (Tanakh: Isaiah 53:4-5)

750 years later the above prophecy by Isaiah was fulfilled by Messiah Jesus.

"When evening came, they brought to him many possessed with demons. He cast out the spirits with a

word, and healed all who were sick; that it might be fulfilled which was spoken through Isaiah the prophet, saying: "He took our infirmities, and bore our diseases." (Brit Chadashah: Mattiyahu [Matthew] 8:16-17)

Yes, my friend, you can BELIEVE God's promises for YOU. **The PURPOSES of the promises of God are for their FULFILLMENT in YOUR life**. ACT on them by FAITH. And by His stripes, you will be—*you have been*—healed.

~ CHAPTER TWENTY-EIGHT ~
HEALING OF RELATIONSHIPS

DESCRIPTION

We need to build relationships by telling people what God has done for us. Be a bridge builder ... not a bridge burner. This chapter covers the causes of bridge burning (breaking of relationships) and healing of the same.

As in football, basketball, baseball, rugby, or any sport ... our best defense is a good offense! **Build relationships with other people ... don't burn them!** Rabbi Shaul (the Apostle Paul) was constantly building good, permanent relationships by leading people to Messiah and by training them to be consistent followers of the Lord.

We need to build relationships by telling people what God has done for us. I know some rabbis and ministers who go a whole day never telling anyone about Messiah

... and then use the excuse that their job is only to equip their followers.

QUESTION: How can you equip the people in your synagogue or church without telling them HOW to share their faith. Some would answer: *"My faith is a private matter."* That is foolishness (unless you're ashamed of your faith). Yeshua taught:

"Whosoever therefore shall confess me before men, him will I confess also before my Father which is in heaven. But whosoever shall deny me before men, him will I also deny before my Father which is in heaven." (Brit Chadashah: Mattiyahu (Mathew) 10:32-33)

"Whosoever therefore shall be ashamed of me and of my words in this adulterous and sinful generation; of him also shall the Son of man be ashamed, when he cometh in the glory of his Father with the holy angels." (Matthew 8:38)

Think of it this way: If something GREAT happens to you, do you keep it private? No! You tell people about it; especially if they are your friends, or someone you like. The real JOY of life is helping people find eternal life through the Lord Jesus and then helping them to grow and be productive leaders.

Sometimes it is God's will for us to break off relationships, but that is surely NOT the case all the time! **If you have a problem constantly breaking off relationships with people, then ask God for healing**.

Usually such problems arise out of insecurity or out of **fear of failure to handle situations**. Insecurity that is usually embedded from childhood; fear of failure resulting from repeated past negative performance. Also, the problems may occur **sometimes** because of a bad spirit (a demon) and must be dealt with by prayer, confession of the Word of God, and sometimes counseling accompanied by exorcism.

Remember, **with Messiah Jesus you have a new start every day**. Learn to cultivate good friendships with people. Show them—and yourself—that the Holy Spirit lives in you.

King Saul was a classic case of a **bridge burner**. King David was a classic case of a **bridge builder**. [1 Samuel Chapters 10 through 31] **Bridge burning usually results from insecurity, fear, or jealousy ... or a**

combination of them; and often manifests with **the OLD order trying to spear the NEW order to the wall.** King Saul was jealous of the anointing from God upon David. He was mad at David and afraid of him because God was with him. (1 Samuel 18:5-12)

Be aware of something: The **new order** does not necessarily mean young in age or seniority ... or inexperienced. The new order can be older people—seasoned, experienced people—breaking away from established form: form that was once fresh with the Spirit.

If we find ourselves in the **old order**, we need to **build bridges with the new order** to establish UNITY for the Lord's sake. This will accomplish two things:

1. It will assure that we are open to what the Spirit is doing; and,

2. It will place us in a position of blessing to receive a new anointing, and to receive God's best as a **peacemaker** for unity's sake [Matthew 5:9]). This way we maintain a position in an OPEN SYSTEM.

Maybe you have had a problem with this in the past ... or maybe you are having a problem with this NOW. **Your** situation may be one where a person is angry with you ... maybe rightfully so, or maybe wrongfully. Well, I've got good news for you. **It's turn around time.** Here is a promise you can claim:

"Surely the wrath of man shall praise you [God]: and the remainder of wrath you shall restrain." (Psalm 76:10)

Pray and ask God to turn the situation around and make the past anger, or wrath, turn into praise to God. Let the situation PRAISE Him! And then, ask God to RESTRAIN the remainder of the wrath so there will be no more anger. It works; I've used that promise many times.

Two other things that are very important in building bridges, and of which we should be cognizant, are as follows:

- To ACKNOWLEDGE the help and work of those with whom we are associated

- To develop the ability to graciously RECEIVE.

~ CHAPTER TWENTY-NINE ~
THE HOLY SPIRIT IN HEALING

I want to talk to you in this chapter about TOTAL healing in your whole man: your whole being. God wants to heal you spiritually, mentally, physically, materially, socially, financially—in your associations and relationships—in your attitudes and your aptitudes: **total healing for the whole person!** This is what Messiah Jesus purchased for you when He shed His BLOOD on the cross-stake. He is the Perfect Lamb of God who made the one-time FINAL supreme sacrifice for the sins of the world.

Yeshua (Jesus) came—He was sent from God—**to bring healing for the separation between God and man.** When Adam sinned in the Garden, he brought separation between God and man, but Messiah Jesus—God's Son—brought healing for that separation. That's why John the Baptist—when he was in the River Jordan administering the mikvah (baptism) for purification of sins—saw Yeshua in the crowd of people, said *"Behold! The Lamb of God who takes away the sin of the world."*

Of course, he was referring to God's Lamb, and associating Him with first Passover in Egypt. The Children of Israel sacrificed the lamb and put the blood of the lamb upon the door and the death angel passed over the homes of ALL who did this.

Friend, if you have the BLOOD of Messiah Yeshua upon the door of your heart by faith, the death angel will pass over you. The Angel of the LORD will protect you. You don't have to be afraid of death because when you die, if you have the Lord Jesus in your heart through faith, you will go straight to Heaven to be with the God of Abraham, Isaac, and Jacob.

It's amazing how medical science from time to time reveals the truth of scripture. There is a case cited by Dr. Keith Mano in his article titled, **"The Bethsaida Miracle,"** (*National Review*, April 21, 1997) concerning a man named Virgil, who was blind since childhood. After successful eye surgery, he could see; however, Virgil's brain had trouble processing visual details into objects that were recognizable. His wife commented, *"Virgil finally put a tree together; he now knows that the trunk and leaves go together to form a complete unit."*

Notice, if you will read in the New Testament, in Mark Chapter 8, Yeshua placed His hands on a blind man ... and then He asked the man, *"What do you see?"* The man said, *"I see men as trees walking."* Then, Yeshua put his hands on the man again, and after that the man saw clearly. This miracle reflects an aspect of sight that was not understood until recently. Eyes may see, but the brain must also have the ability to assemble the visual images into something meaningful.

Only the the Holy Spirit would have known that in those days; there was NO scientific evidence to reveal that. The Holy Spirit wrote the account of this miracle by inspiration through Mark. **Mark (in his human knowledge) would NOT know that a newly restored sight would see men as trees walking**. And, without the medical knowledge of that day, nobody could have written that account like that. **Only the Spirit of God knew those things: the same spirit of God that raised Messiah Jesus from the dead!**

It's the same Spirit of God, the Ruach Elohim, that will minister the resurrection POWER of Messiah to you today IF you will trust Him. My friend, Jesus loves you ... He gave His own life for you. He came to heal the separation between God and man. And, my friend, **the healing POWER of Messiah is available to you today**. Call upon Him!

The Prophet Jeremiah gives us a PROMISE from the LORD: *"Call unto me, and I will answer you, and show you great and mighty things, which you do NOT know."* (Tanakh: Jeremiah 33:3)

The POWER of the LORD is present to heal you today: spiritually, mentally, physically, materially, socially, and in every other way, shape, or form.

Today is the day of your deliverance!

~ CHAPTER THIRTY ~
YOU CAN BE HEALED TODAY

One area of healing, called FAITH healing, has at its core three (3) prerequisites:

- You have to **WANT** to be healed.

- You have to **KNOW** you can be healed.

- You have to **BELIEVE** you **WILL** be healed.

Remember: you can always pray, *"Lord, I believe. Please, God, help my unbelief."*

God is NOT some mean tyrant. God loves you and that is WHY He has provided healing for you.

*"Praise the LORD, my soul, And **don't forget all his benefits***;

*Who **forgives all your sins***; *Who **heals all your diseases***;

*Who **redeems your life from destruction;** Who crowns you with loving kindness and tender mercies;*

*Who satisfies your desire with good things, So that **your youth is renewed** like the eagle's."* – Psalm 103:2-5

Can you **believe** in God who loves you so much He gave His only Son—the Messiah of Israel—as an atonement, a just compensation, for your sins so that the separation between you and God could be healed?

There is nothing God will not do for you; He already gave the BEST HE had for you.

God does NOT want you to be sick, in pain, or diseased. Sometimes sickness is due to NOT being connected to God ... that is, NOT knowing Him personally. And, lots of times people are sick, in pain, or diseased because of involvement in the occult, or witchcraft, or just plain sin and disobedience. Even so, God is quick to grant forgiveness and healing as we just read in Psalm 103: *"Who **forgives all your sins;** Who **heals all your diseases."***

Messiah's atonement on the cross stake covered ALL sickness: spiritual, mental, and physical. His BLOOD made us WHOLE: it paid for our sins. **It bought us OUT OF the hands of the devil—the enemy of our souls, minds, and bodies—and it bought us UNTO God**. The BLOOD purchased us. We have a rightful citizenship in Heaven and **all we have to do is exercise the rights that pertain to our citizenship**. One of those rights is the ability to call on our Heavenly Father for forgiveness, healing, and help.

Psalm 107:17-21 tells us:

> *"Fools are afflicted because of their disobedience, And because of their iniquities.*
>
> *Their soul abhors all kinds of food. They draw near to the gates of death.*
>
> *Then they cry to Yahweh in their trouble, He saves them out of their distresses.*
>
> ***He sends his word, and heals them***, *And* ***delivers them*** *from their graves.*
>
> *Let them praise Yahweh for his loving kindness, for his wonderful works to the children of men!"*

Trust Him today, my friend.

■ **WANT** to be healed.

■ **KNOW** you can be healed.

■ **BELIEVE** you **WILL** be healed.

Call upon the name of the LORD. **Ask Messiah Jesus to heal you NOW** … ask Him to save you. Psalm 50:15 says, *"Call upon Me in the day of trouble: I will deliver you."*

~ CHAPTER THIRTY-ONE ~
HEALING OF EMOTIONAL WOUNDS

There is nothing more vexing to the people I have counseled through the years than emotional hurt, or to put it simply: **a broken heart**. People can have physical, even mental disease, and sometimes compensate for them in their own way. However, wounds of the emotions (for example, a broken heart, rejection, scorn) are not only difficult to assess, but can elude instant deliverance.

In the Hebrew Tanakh (the Old Covenant scriptures) we read: *"A man's spirit will sustain him in sickness, But a crushed spirit, who can bear?"* (Proverbs 18:14) Another translation reads: *"The spirit of a man will sustain his infirmity; but a wounded spirit who can bear?"* The scripture is informing us that a crushed or wounded spirit is a burden almost too heavy for an individual to bear.

Realize that the primal cause of this attack against your emotions—your spirit—was not the person or people who offended you. **It was the devil (Satan) that used**

them. The enemy of your soul is NEVER fair, and NEVER honest. He likes to hurt people and lie to them. He likes to kick you when you are down.

That's WHY you need to take your authority SOON after the attack(s) against you. The enemy (Satan) knows that if he can wound your spirit you will be defeated if you do not take decisive AND immediate action. If you have been baptized in the Holy Spirit, **power pray** in tongues and break the attack of the wicked one against you.

The scar over your wounded spirit will develop to the place of shielding the wound, thus serving two (2) purposes:

- **Protecting** it from future attacks, hurts, and vulnerability; and,

- **Disguising it**—camouflaging it—hiding it from view.

The enemy of your soul does not care HOW he achieves this wound: through personal loss (material loss or the loss of a loved one), through demons, through mental assaults, through a friend, through a relative, through a religious person, or thru an immoral person. No one is perfect; therefore, even a person who lives a normally holy life may have a moment where he / she slips and attacks another person verbally or in gossip or in behavior.

A person can also be wounded emotionally through discouragement of any kind ... possibly the result of a friend or loved one going astray.

WHAT IS THE ANSWER?

There are **two things** you must do:

FIRST, Rise up and take your authority over this attack. No matter WHAT the cause of your hurt, it is an attack from the enemy of your soul: Satan, the devil. Even if it was another person (which it usually is) that caused your spirit (your emotions) to be wounded, the source is the devil: he hates you. The other person may not even know they have done you wrong. On the other hand, they may have wanted to do you wrong. **In either case, they unwittingly were pawns in the hands of the devil.**

The scriptures tell us: *"The thief [the devil] only comes to steal, to kill, and to destroy."* *"[Jesus said] I came that they may have life, and that they may have it abundantly.*

I am the good shepherd. The good shepherd lays down his life for the sheep." – John 10:10-11

SECOND, forgive the person or people who offended you. This is tough to do, but you have to do it. Otherwise, they are preventing or hindering your healing and deliverance from the wound(s) you have experienced. Since they have already caused you enough trouble, why would you let them bother you anymore?! **Release them (by forgiving them) so you will NOT be tied to them (bound to them) any longer.**

The scriptures also tell us: *"And be kind to one another, tenderhearted, forgiving each other, just as God also in Messiah Jesus forgave you."* – Ephesians 4:32

DO IT NOW

FIRST: In the name of Messiah Jesus, bind the devil (Satan) and break his hold upon you that was caused from the emotional wounds you received.

SECOND: PRAY and tell God you forgive the person, or the people, who have wounded you. Release them into the hands of God, who has told us:

■ *"**To me belongs vengeance**, and recompence; their foot shall slide in due time ..."*

■ *"Dearly beloved, avenge not yourselves, but rather give place unto wrath: for it is written, **'Vengeance is mine; I will repay'**, says the Lord."*

I know this teaching is going to help you, my friend.

~ CHAPTER THIRTY-TWO ~
MIRACLES
HOW TO KNOW REAL FROM FALSE

Supernatural occurrences, or wonders, that happen as a result of God intervening in the affairs of man are MIRACLES. These are extra-natural happenings, outside the realm of man's natural, earthly, experiences.

MIRACLES as when Elisha, the man of God, made the metal axe head swim which was lost in the water (2 Kings 6:1-7). Or, when Elijah raised the widow's son from the dead (1 Kings 17:17-23), not to mention the many miracles of healing, deliverance, and provision in both the Old Testament (Tanakh) and New Testament (Brit Chadashah) of the Holy Bible.

Not everything that appears to be a miracle is from God. Just as in Moses' day there were magicians who did lying wonders, so there are today. The Holy Bible tells us that in the last days the coming world ruler—the false-Messiah or the beast—will have his false prophet perform seeming miracles.

Many times, people are drawn into false religions and into witchcraft because they think they have evidenced or received a miracle. For example, at times Satan may have his demon spirits **afflict a person** with sickness or disease. If the person goes to a New Age healer, or someone in the dark works of the devil, it may APPEAR that they have been healed.

What has happened is simply this: the demons withdrew their affliction, and so it appeared the person was healed. However, because the sick person submitted themselves to the "channel" or person being used by Satan (such as a New Age practitioner, Reiki practitioner, or an occult spirit medium) for prayer—like a false minister, a shaman, practitioner, psychic, or witch —they then end up usually in a worse state. That is, the same and/or other demons then take them over. (Matthew 12:45 / Luke 11:26)

Real miracles, however—God's MIRACLES—always glorify the LORD: the Holy One of Israel. **The Holy Spirit is God's agent on earth to supply the resurrection POWER of Messiah Jesus**, and He will always magnify Jesus—the Son of God—who came to earth in human flesh.

Do you, or does someone you know, need a miracle today? There is nothing too hard for the Lord. Trust his love for you! *"Behold, I am the LORD, the God of all flesh: is there any thing too hard for me?"* (Tanakh: Jeremiah 32:27)

We have received many testimonies in the mail from Muslims who have been healed when receiving Messiah Jesus as LORD. **Nothing is too hard for the LORD!** It's amazing that MOST of these testimonies are from Muslims who received Yeshua (Jesus) AFTER he healed them and they had a revelation of WHO Messiah is. They then renounced Islam as a false religion and Mohammed as a false prophet. Messiah Yeshua is ALIVE to help you today. **Ask him for your miracle!**

~ CHAPTER THIRTY-THREE ~
HEALING FROM CLAUSTROPHOBIA

Do you ever feel like you're shut in: by air? by water? by situation?

Or, do you ever feel like you're not breathing fast enough?

Although most medical journals and resources discriminate to a degree between claustrophobia and anxiety (or panic attacks), there is a highly positive correlation between the two classifications of disorders.

When we speak of disorder, we are speaking of a condition out of the norm. So, a perfectly sane person can have these disorders, just as a perfectly mentally competent person may have a tooth ache.

Claustrophobia is one of the most common phobias in America. Claustrophobia is characterized by panic that is a result of being in enclosed spaces. This panic is activated by an irrational fear of a certain situation. **The situation may be real or imagined**. It may be physical or psychological; and it may be spiritual, that is, demoniacal.

The important thing to realize is that—no matter what the source—claustrophobia can be overcome ... and complete deliverance effected.

Lots of people mistake claustrophobia for anxiety attacks. The common denominator in claustrophobic incidences is the feeling of containment: *"I'm stuck; I have to get out of here,"* ... or *"I have to get away from this situation." "I do not have control; something ... or someone ... has control of me."*

Lots of times, minor psychological claustrophobic attacks happen at night when a person is either asleep or has been sleeping. However, there is a "sector" of these types of attacks which happen as a result of demonic activity initiated through the avenue of dreams or subconscious activity.

Most medical resources assert that there is NO cure for claustrophobia, but that there are several forms of treatment that can alleviate the situation.

But I have some GOOD NEWS for you: **there is nothing ... and no one ... that God can not heal.**

If you need healing ... or deliverance ... from claustrophobia, do the following:

- Ask God to give you discernment over the situation before it happens and during the occurrence.

- Realize that this situation is triggered by either an internal (inside yourself) or external (condition or assault outside yourself) source.

- Believe that YOU have the POWER, with God's help, to overcome this situation.

- Pray, and call on the name of Yeshua (Jesus) to help you. Cry out to Him. Ask Him to help you.

- Speak (declare) the BLOOD of Messiah (Christ) **over yourself** and **against Satan and demons** that are trying to amplify the situation in your mind and spirit. Say this: *"I declare the BLOOD of Messiah (Christ) over me and against this situation."*

- Then, bind Satan and his demons in the name of Yeshua (Jesus) and command them to leave. Just say this to the devil: *"I bind you Satan and your demons in the name of Jesus the Messiah and command you to leave. The LORD rebuke you."*

■ Start praising God in tongues, the language of the the Holy Spirit. If you don't know HOW to do this, study the book by Prince Handley titled *How to Receive the Power of God with Gifts of the Spirit.*

I trust this teaching has helped you.

~ CHAPTER THIRTY-FOUR ~
HEALING OF JOINT
AND BONE PAIN

Somebody reading this message has pain in your joints and bones. By the time you are finished reading this message, God will heal you.

The healing power of Messiah (Christ) is coming to you. You have been miserable, but Jesus (Yeshua) is going to bring you comfort.

There are several causes of joint and pain discomfort:

Poor nutrition

Try calcium and vitamin D-rich recipes. **If your body lacks calcium, it takes it from bones. Vitamin D helps your body absorb calcium**. Make sure you are getting enough protein. Protein is an important building block of bones, muscles, cartilage, skin, and blood, and also necessary for repair. However, beware of high protein diet over a long period of time. Salt is a major culprit in depriving the body of calcium. The more salt you eat, the more calcium gets carried away by urine.

It may be difficult to get adequate calcium from food if you don't eat dairy. Osteoporosis experts do say the best source of calcium is from foods, not supplements. Food contains important nutrients that help the body utilize calcium.

Envy

The Bible tells us: *"A sound heart is the life of the flesh: but envy the rottenness of the bones."* (Proverbs 14:30) Envy, or jealousy, will produce destruction in your bones. This is a spiritual law. Just as gravity is a determined law of the universe, so is envy. If you have a problem with envy, then stop right NOW and ask God to forgive you. (At the same time, forgive others.)

Lack of (proper) exercise

Exercise more to decrease pain and feel more energetic? Does that sound paradoxical? Not so ... it's true. Regular exercise helps reverse joint stiffness, builds muscle, and boosts overall fitness. But check with your doctor first before starting an exercise regimen. To derive the most advantage from a bone-builidng diet,

163

you'll want to do regular weight-bearing exercise. This includes any activity that uses the weight of your body or outside weights to stress the bones and muscles.

Osteoporosis

Thinning bones is a serious condition that can result in tremendous pain with fractures. Prevention and treatment of osteoporosis include calcium and vitamin D, regular exercise, and osteoporosis medications, if needed.

Rheumatoid arthritis

A chronic type of arthritis. RA is an autoimmune disease in which the immune system mistakenly attacks normal tissues in the body, causing inflammation. The result is pain, stiffness, and swelling in the joints.

Early symptoms of RA include fatigue, joint pain, and stiffness. Early and effective rheumatoid arthritis treatment can improve the prognosis and may help prevent joint and bone destruction associated with RA.

Atrophication

Atrophication is a wasting away or progressive decline, basically degeneration. It is the tendency to atrophy and degrade over periods of time due to lack of usage or practice.

Atrophy is the partial or complete wasting away of a part of the body. Causes of atrophy include poor nourishment, poor circulation, loss of hormonal support, loss of nerve supply to the target organ, disuse or lack of exercise or disease intrinsic to the tissue itself. Hormonal and nerve inputs that maintain an organ or body part are referred to as trophic.

Atrophy is a general physiological process of reabsorption and breakdown of tissues, involving apoptosis on a cellular level. When it occurs as a result of disease or loss of trophic support due to other disease, it is termed pathological atrophy, although it can be a part of normal body development and homeostasis as well.

So with the information we have discussed in mind, begin to write a NEW slate for your lifestyle. Make some changes.

To help you get a NEW start for healing and relief from joint and bone pain, remember God's promise to YOU:

"Behold, I am the LORD, the God of all flesh: is there any thing too hard for me?" (Tanakh: Jeremiah 32:27)

~ *CHAPTER THIRTY-FIVE* ~

HOW TO BE HEALED AT HOLY COMMUNION AND PASSOVER

DESCRIPTION

We should expect MIRACLES during Communion and during Passover. I received an instant MIRACLE during Passover Seder at synagogue. Great pain and misery resulting from several rare diseases I developed in Africa that could not be diagnosed medically were healed instantly.

You must know that healing belongs to you. There is no need for you to depart from health.

You can be healed ... walk in health ... and help others to do the same.

In this chapter I want to teach you **HOW to be healed by HOLY COMMUNION** (the Lord's Supper, or Eucharist) **and**, also, by celebrating **PASSOVER**.

167

We should expect MIRACLES during the Holy Communion (the Lord's Supper) and, also, during Passover. We are celebrating what Messiah did FOR US, and he told us to do this in order to remember Him until he returns. *"For as often as you eat this bread, and drink this cup, you SHOW the Lord's death until he comes [again]."* [1 Corinthians 11:26]

The Holy Bible teaches us in the 1 Corinthians 11:27-32 of the Brit Chadasha (the New Testament, or Covenant) that we are to do **two things** when we come to the Lord's Supper:

Discern the Lord's body; and,

Examine ourselves.

To **discern** means **to see His sacrifice for us as "distinct" from other things**. See his body (the bread) beaten—even before the cross—as the Roman soldiers whip (or, flog) him, leaving his back bruised and **striped** with open wounds. See his head **pierced** by the crown of thorns, causing blood to flow down his face and chest. And then ... see his hands and feet nailed with rough spikes to the wooden cross. All of this **for us ...** and **for God**!

This is why the Pesach bread, the matzo, has pin holes and stripes. At Passover, we are celebrating deliverance from bondage in Egypt ... and, also, spiritual bondage; and drink the RED WINE (or juice) to commemorate the RED BLOOD Messiah shed for us as **the Lamb of God**, without fault or blemish, who takes away the sin of the world. This is why the matzo bread has pin holes and stripes. The early Messianic believers added this to the Passover. Almost all the early Messianic believers in Yeshua (Jesus) were Jewish.

When we drink of the cup, we see his blood shed for us: sinless blood, having good credit in the bank of Heaven. Not blood which inherited sin from Adam and his race, but **blood from a miracle birth** from above: as the Spirit of God breathed on the womb of a virgin, creating NEW LIFE from God.

> *"In whom we have redemption THROUGH HIS BLOOD, the forgiveness of sins, according to the riches of his grace."* (Brit Chadashah: Ephesians 1:7)

> *"For the life of the flesh is in the blood: and I have given it to you upon the altar to make an atonement for your souls: for it is the blood that*

makes an atonement for the soul." (Torah: Leviticus 17:11)

"So Messiah was once offered to bear the sins of many." (Brit Chadashah Hebrew 9:28)

Yeshua's body and mind bore the punishment for **our** sins ... his blood paid the PRICE to redeem, or ransom, **us**. And God raised him from the dead: **Yeshua is ALIVE to save and to heal you!** Yes, miracles and healing are available in the Holy Communion and the Passover by discerning the Lord's body ... seeing him and what he did for us. Isaiah Chapter 53 in the Tanach tells us:

He bore **our** sicknesses and diseases.

He carried (away) **our** pains.

He was wounded and bruised for **our** sin.

The LORD laid on him the sin of **us all**.

And with his *stripes* **WE ARE HEALED.**

~ CHAPTER THIRTY-SIX ~
HEALING FROM ANXIETY
AND PANIC ATTACKS

In Chapter 26 we discussed "Healing from Stress." Anxiety is a normal reaction to stress. It may help a person to deal with a difficult situation, for example at work or at school, by causing one to cope with it, or to confront another person or situation. However, **when anxiety becomes excessive**, it may fall under the classification of an **anxiety disorder**. There are several types of anxiety disorder:

■ Generalized anxiety disorder

■ Obsessive-Compulsive Disorder

■ Panic Disorder

■ Panic Intense Stress Syndrome

■ Post-Traumatic Stress Disorder

■ Social Phobia or, Social Anxiety Disorder

- Developmental External Manic Oppressive Neurosis

The latter case deals in the area of demonic oppression or possession, an area not clearly defined by medical science, but fairly well known to most experienced psychotherapists. In practice—for complete deliverance of the subject—it should be the domain of only experienced Holy Spirit anointed Messianic rabbis or ministers of the Gospel.

Of all the types mentioned, there is an area of commonality, a Boolean center if you will, that manifests itself—to whatever degree, or spectral terminus—in anxiety.

Anxiety can be a psychological or physiological state characterized by components that may combine to cause an **unpleasant feeling associated with fear, worry, or uneasiness**. In this study we will address the **behavioral** aspects of anxiety: particularly the **actions or reactions**. For material dealing with healing of emotions," consult Chapter 31: "Healing of Emotional Wounds."

The basal causations of anxiety are fear and worry. They play upon each other. They feed each other and escalate each other. Fear exacerbates worry, and worry exacerbates fear. They are congruous and meld together as **concern**. After the cycle is replete, they become synonymous as **generic fear**. **The resultant effect produced is the product of anxiety.**

The Bible tells us: *"For God has **not given us the spirit of fear**; but of power, and of love, and of a sound mind."* (2 Timothy 1:7) The original language for the term **sound mind** (*sophronismo*s) gives the meaning: **"discipline; self control."** If you know the LORD, you have NOT received a spirit of fear; but you have received by the Spirit of God a spirit of **power, love, and of self control**.

Fear is a spirit. God is love, and God is a spirit. The Bible informs us the, *"Perfect love casts out all fear."* **Love is therefore greater than fear**. That is WHY the scripture explains to us: *"Whoever fears is NOT made **perfect** in love."* Can you SEE the POWER here? **Perfect love casts out fear**. It **commands** fear to leave: to depart. **Since fear is a spirit, you can speak to it**. Command fear, in the name of Yeshua (or, Jesus), to depart.

It is interesting to note that the talmidim of Yeshua came back after a trip he sent them on, and declared, *"Rabbi, even the demons are subject to us in your name!"* Then, Yeshua answered them, saying, *"Rejoice not that the demons are subject to you in my name, but rather that YOUR NAMES are written down in Heaven!"*

If you are afraid of **someone**, ask God to give you LOVE for them. If you are afraid of **something** bind it in the name of Jesus—*through prayer or verbal command*—and command it to leave. That is, command the spirit behind the thing(s) you fear to leave—to depart—in the name of Jesus. Oh, they may TRY to come back at times, but **all you have to do** is be dictatorial in the name of Messiah Jesus. Take your God given authority in the name of Yeshua (Jesus). [*"Yeshua" is the Hebrew name for Jesus.*]

The scripture encourages us as follows:

> *"You will keep him in **perfect peace** whose mind is fixed on You, because he trusts in You."* – Isaiah 26:3

> *"**Have no anxiety** [or, worry] about anything, but in everything by prayer and supplication **with***

thanksgiving *let your requests be made known to God."* – Philippians 4:6

If you are NOT sure that you know the Messiah of Israel personally, **pray this prayer**:

> *"God of Abraham, Isaac, and Jacob, if Yeshua is really my Messiah, then reveal Him to me."*

When he reveals Him, my friend, then pray to Him and ASK Him WHAT He wants you to do.

~ CHAPTER THIRTY-SEVEN ~
HOW TO BE HEALED BY
LAYING ON OF HANDS

Jesus healed the separation between God and man through his work FOR US, and therefore ended Satan's dominion over ALL who would trust in Christ! *"For this purpose the Son of God was manifested, that he might DESTROY the works of the devil."* [1 John 3:8]

Jesus "carried" sickness, sin, disease, poverty, and oppression—the works of the devil (Satan)—FOR YOU. **You don't have to carry them any longer.** They do NOT belong to the believer in Christ!

WHAT JESUS DID FOR YOU
YOU DON'T HAVE TO DO!

Now that you know that physical and mental healing belong to the believer in Christ—as much as spiritual healing—you need to know how to obtain it: HOW TO BE HEALED! There are several ways, or avenues, to obtain AND to minister Christ's healing power. They are listed below:

■ THE WORD OF GOD

■ LAYING ON OF HANDS

■ HOLY COMMUNION

■ ANOINTING WITH OIL

■ PRAYER & PROPER MENTAL ATTITUDE

In Chapter 11 we discussed how to be healed by the Word of God.

In this chapter I am going to teach you how to be healed by **the laying on of hands.**

LAYING ON OF HANDS

After Jesus Christ was raised from the dead and before he went back to Heaven, he said:

> *"And these signs shall follow them that believe; in my name shall they cast out devils; they shall speak with new tongues ... they shall lay hands on the sick, and they shall recover."* (Mark 16:17-18)

Notice three things Jesus told us:

"In my name ..."

"you shall lay hands on the sick,"

"they (the sick) shall recover."

IN MY NAME – It is **the name of Jesus the Messiah**, (the Holy One of God) which is to accompany the laying on of hands. It is THE NAME that is above every name [Philippians 2:8-9]. **The NAME of Jesus Christ joins God's power to your action.**

The name of Jesus identifies you: it tells "sickness" and "demons" the authority behind your action and command. It tells them you belong to and are a believer in Jesus the Messiah: the One who conquered them and their master, Satan! The name of Jesus identifies you with the One who CREATED the world and who BOUGHT IT BACK (after Adam's sin) with his own blood!

Use the name of Jesus with authority: as a citizen of Messiah's Kingdom. If you are in doubt, just whisper the name of Jesus for a while: *"Jesus, Jesus, Jesus ...."* It will call God's power to the scene! If it is a case of demon affliction, speak with authority (not your authority, but Christ's) and say: *"You devil, come out! I command*

178

you in the name of Jesus Christ to come out of this person!"

YOU SHALL LAY HANDS ON THE SICK - If you are a believer in Jesus, then God wants to use you to heal others. You have the privilege—as well as the responsibility—of laying hands on the sick and praying for them: whether they are Christians or non-Christians. (See Luke 4:40; Acts 28:8.)

Your hands become Christ's hands: his tool! The power of the Holy Spirit flows through your hands. You may not see it ... you may not feel it ... but it is POWER just the same. The devil is afraid of your touch! Because of distance, sometimes, you are not able to lay hands on the sick person. (The person you want to pray for may be in a different city or country.) You can then **send them a "prayer cloth" to be laid on the body of the sick person**.

"And God wrought special miracles by the hands of Paul: so that from his body were brought unto the sick handkerchiefs or aprons, and the diseases departed from them, and the evil spirits went out of them." (Acts 19:11-12)

179

Prayer cloths are very effective! Demons (evil spirits) are cast out, sick bodies are healed, minds are restored. **Pray over the cloth (lay your hands on it) in the name of Jesus Christ and ask God to send deliverance, healing, and blessing**.

If you are a Christian, you have more POWER than the devil ever hoped to have! Satan is afraid of your handkerchief!!

THEY SHALL RECOVER - Forget what your mind or eyes tell you. Believe what God says. You may not see the person you pray for be healed as soon as you think you should ... however, you may see them be healed instantly. The important thing is to KNOW that they will recover. Note: In some cases the sick person may be hindering their own healing; such cases will be covered later in this book in Chapter 40: *"Healing Through Proper Mental Attitude"*.

The Holy Spirit is God's agent on earth to supply the healing power of Christ. Whether the sick person is healed instantly or over a period of time—whether they feel God's power or not—Jesus promised, *"These signs shall follow them that believe ... in My name ... they shall lay hands on the sick, and they [the sick] shall* *recover."* Your job is to serve **by faith** in obedience to Christ's command: **"You go ... they shall recover."** Read again Mark 16:15-18 and notice the command and the promise!

~ CHAPTER THIRTY-EIGHT ~
PHYSICAL, MENTAL AND
SPIRITUAL HEALING FOR YOU

In a previous chapter we saw that **spiritual** death—SEPARATION FROM GOD—which produced physical sickness and disease—and the death of the body—HAD TO BE HEALED! This is why God sent his only Son, Jesus the Messiah, to earth.

> "For as by one man's disobedience many were made sinners, **so by the obedience of one** [Jesus] shall many be made righteous." (Romans 5:19)

In Isaiah Chapter 53 we see just **what** Yeshua did ... **why** he came to earth!

> "Surely He has borne **our** sicknesses and diseases, and carried [away] **our** pains; yet we did esteem Him stricken, smitten of God and afflicted. (Verse 4)

*But He was wounded for **our** transgressions, he was bruised for **our** iniquities: the chastisement of **our** peace was upon Him; and **with His stripes [bruises] we are healed**.*" (Verse 5)

All we like sheep have gone astray; we have turned every one to his own way, and the LORD has laid on Him the iniquity [or, sin] of us all." (Verse 6)

What Isaiah prophesied in the Old Testament [Tanakh] **was fulfilled 750 years later** by the Messiah of Israel, Yeshua HaMaschiach (Jesus the "Christ," or the "**Anointed One**"). He bore **our** sicknesses and diseases. He carried away **our** pains. He was wounded and bruised for **our** sin; the LORD laid on Him the sin of us all. And with His stripes **we** are healed.

In some Bibles Isaiah 53:4 reads: *"Surely he has borne our **griefs** and carried our **sorrows**."* However, the original Hebrew (the original language of the Old Testament) for the words "grief" and "sorrow" is "**choli**" and "**macob**", respectively. "**Choli**" means "**sickness and disease**". "**Macob**" means "**pain**" ... **acute pain; intense suffering: mental or physical**.

To prove that Isaiah meant in this passage that healing would be included in Messiah's work for us, we need only to consult the Brit Chadashah (New Testament) record of Yeshua's ministry in Mattiyahu (Matthew) Chapter 8, verses 16-17:

> *"When the evening was come, they brought unto Him many that were possessed with devils; and He cast out the spirits with his word, and healed ALL that were sick.*
>
> *That it might be fulfilled which was spoken by Isaiah the prophet, saying, 'Himself [Jesus the Messiah] took our infirmities, and bore our sicknesses'."*

Jesus fulfilled what Isaiah the prophet said 750 years before:

- He bore **our** sicknesses and diseases.

- He carried away **our** pains.

- With his stripes **WE ARE HEALED**.

Yeshua's body and mind took punishment for **us** ... his blood paid for **our** sins. His body was beaten, wounded, and bruised (even before he was crucified) and then he was nailed to the wooden cross ... FOR **OUR** HEALING: **spiritual, physical, and mental!**

Be healed in the Name of Jesus ... then go heal others!

~ CHAPTER THIRTY-NINE ~
HEALING BY ANOINTING WITH OIL

DESCRIPTION

You can be healed by either the elders of the synagogue or the church anointing you with oil in The Name of the LORD. There are hindrances to healing that sometimes must be dealt with and in this chapter we discuss them, also.

ANOINTING WITH OIL

In the Holy Bible, anointing with oil is representative of the ministry of the Spirit of God. Oil is a "type"—it represents the Holy Spirit. In James 5:14-15 in the Brit Chadasha (New Testament) we read:

> "Is any sick among you? Let him call for the elders of the church; and let them pray over him, anointing him with oil in the name of the Lord.

And the prayer of faith shall save the sick, and the Lord shall raise him up; and if he has committed sins, they shall be forgiven him."

It is the name of **Jesus**, *the Messiah*, accompanied by the anointing with oil and the prayer of faith that will bring your healing.

Notice, that it is "the prayer of faith" ... NOT a medicinal rubdown. And it must be connected to the Name of Jesus. Also, to prove that it is NOT a massage or rubdown—but a spiritual act accompanied in partnership with the Holy Spirit—if the peron has committed sins, they shall be forgiven. No "rubdown" or massage can forgive sins!

There is **another type of anointing with oil** which may be referred to as "evangelistic" anointing. It is just as much a part of evangelistic ministry as preaching, or teaching, or winning people to Messiah. It does not require the sick person to "call" for the elders of the synagogue church; nor is it only for Messianic believers. Mark 6:12-13 tells us:

"And they went out, and preached that men should repent. And they cast out many devils,

and ANOINTED WITH OIL many that were sick, and healed them. "

Carry a bottle of anointing oil with you at all times, ready for use. Let God use you to heal others.

HINDRANCES TO HEALING

Your mind—and therefore your body—can be abused by many things. At times there are hindrances to healing: things or conditions that are causing the sickness or affliction, and that must be dealt with before healing can take place permanently. Things such as:

■ Unforgiveness, bitterness, or resentment (Mark 11:25-26)

■ Envy and strife (James 3:16)

■ Improper food, rest, sunshine, or exercise (Isaiah 30:15)

■ Speaking evil of, or causing harm to, God's ministers (1 Samuel 26:9)

■ Involvement in the occult or in witchcraft (Deuteronomy 18:10-12)

■ Association with religious cults (1 John 4:1-3 / 1 John 5:20)

Whether sickness is caused by disobeying God through an unforgiving spirit, strife, or resentment ... involvement in the occult ... or association with religious cults ... **Jesus the Anointed One is the answer!**

Through prayer we can come to God and ask Him to **forgive** us of all these things; we can also ask Him to **deliver** us, if necessary! 1 John 1:9 says, *"If we confess our sins, he is faithful and just to forgive us our sins, and to cleanse us from all unrighteousness."* In Psalm 50:15 we read, *"Call upon me in the day of trouble: I will deliver you, and you shall glorify me."*

~ CHAPTER FORTY ~
HEALING THROUGH PROPER
MENTAL ATTITUDE

DESCRIPTION

Satan is a **destroyer**, who causes sickness and disease. God is a **healer**, and **God calls sickness captivity**. The devil came to "steal from you, kill you, and destroy you," but Yeshua (Jesus) came to "bring you LIFE ... and life more abundantly." Learn HOW Job, who lost everything he had (including his health), was healed.

———————

We see the importance of proper mental attitude in the life of Job. Job was afflicted by Satan with sore boils from his feet to his head. Also, the devil destroyed Job's wealth and killed his seven sons and three daughters. Job's experience was a rare, "once-in-the-Bible" case. It was allowed by God to prove that a certain man ("greatest of all the men in the east") would not curse God even if he lost everything, including his health.

It shows that **Satan is a "destroyer," who causes sickness and disease.** It shows that **God is a "healer," and that God calls sickness "captivity."** Job was a just man; even God said so. His experience presents a question that many people ask: **"Why?" Notice seven things:**

1. Job's case was unique; it was NOT an example! Don't use it as an excuse to be sick.

2. Satan accused Job of serving God only because of God's blessing, protection and help.

3. Satan is the one—the Bible says—who STOLE Job's health, KILLED his children, and DESTROYED his property. (Job, Chapters 1 and 2; Also, see John 10:10)

4. Job proved faithful in trial. Job did not sin with his lips or charge God foolishly. (Job 1:22 and 2:10)

5. The Bible calls Job's sickness and loss "captivity." (Job 42:10). Yeshua said, *"If the Son shall make you free, you shall be free indeed."* (John 8:36)

6. Job was healed! Because of proper mental attitude, Job prayed for his friends (who were not real friends); this was when God delivered Job. (Job 42:10)

7. *"The Lord gave Job twice as much as he had before." "The Lord blessed the latter end of Job more than his beginning."* (Job 42:10-12)

Even though Job lived on the other side of the cross stake (that is, **before** Messiah's atonement for us)—not having the advantages of Messiah's work and authority over Satan as we do—he was still healed through prayer and proper mental attitude. A **proper mental attitude** will cause you to have an instinctive reaction to sickness and ill-health: you will **refuse it ...** knowing it does NOT belong to you!

You will speak to sickness, saying, *"Sickness, I resist you in the name of Jesus the Messiah by whose stripes I am healed."* Notice two things. You resisted the sickness by: **1**. Speaking to it; and, **2**. Using scripture (the Word of God).

The Holy Bible says in James 4:7 *"Resist the devil, and he will flee from you."* In Matthew 4:11, we see how

Jesus Christ resisted Satan. He did it the same way you are to do it: with the Word of God. Each time Jesus spoke to the devil, Jesus said, *"It is written ..."*

It's interesting to note that each time Yeshua quoted the word of God to Satan it was from the Torah in the Book of Deuteronomy. This is the first book that was attacked in the late 1800's by so called higher criticism and questioning its textual integrity. Satan hates the Book of Deuteronomy, as he does the Torah ... and ALL of God's Holy Word.

Proper nutrition, rest, sunshine, and exercise are all beneficial to a proper mental attitude and maintenance of good health. **Scriptural fasting and honoring the LORD's Day**—or Sabbath—**contribute, also, to a proper mental attitude**; and are laws of God with **built-in bonuses of health and blessing**. Read Isaiah Chapter 58 in the Tanakh (Old Testament).

Isaiah the Prophet told 750 years before how **Messiah would come and be the sacrificed Lamb of God, and by whose stripes on the cross stake we would be healed**. (Tanakh – Isaiah Chapter 53)

Now ... **you** can be healed. If you want to meet the Healer, Jesus the Anointed One, **NOW** is the time! Invite God's Son, Yeshua, to come into your life by praying this prayer:

"Lord Jesus, I know that you are The Great Physician. You loved me enough to shed your sinless blood and die for me on the cross stake that I might be healed. I know you are alive. Please forgive my sins, come into my life and be my Messiah. Help me to live for you, and take me to Heaven when I die."

If you prayed that prayer and meant it, then you have eternal life and your sins are ALL forgiven. You have been healed in your spirit. Know that God has heard and answered your prayer! The Bible says, *"Whoever shall call upon the name of the Lord shall be saved."* [Romans 10:13.] Notice, God did NOT say "may be saved" ... "might be saved" ... or even "probably," but his promise is: **"Whoever will call ... WILL BE saved!"**

~ CHAPTER FORTY-ONE ~
HEALING FROM THE
ATTACKS OF SATAN

The devil (Satan) wants to hurt you and make you sick. Yeshua (Jesus) wants to heal you and make you whole.

God sent his Son, Yeshua, to earth to heal the separation between God and man. You can be healed in body, mind, and spirit.

Read and meditate on the following Scriptures. Your inner man—your human spirit—will then be built up AND faith will arise for your healing. *"So then **faith** comes **by hearing**, and **hearing by** the Word of God."* – Romans 10:17

**THE DEVIL WANTS TO HURT YOU
AND MAKE YOU SICK**
The thief (Satan) comes ... to steal, and to kill, and to destroy.
(John 10:10)

YESHUA WANTS TO HELP YOU
AND MAKE YOU WHOLE
I am come that they might have life ... abundantly.
(John 10:10)

YESHUA WILL GIVE YOU
POWER OVER THE DEVIL
I give you power ... over all the power of the
enemy.
(Luke 10:19)

CONTINUE TO TRUST ONLY MESSIAH
AS YOUR LORD - TURN FROM SIN
Stop sinning, so that nothing worse may happen to
you.
(John 5:14)

DO NOT RECEIVE SICKNESS OR PAIN
Resist the devil, and he will flee from you.
(James 4:7)

RESIST SATAN AND HIS WORKS
BY SPEAKING GOD'S WORD
Yeshua said unto him (the devil), 'It is written ...'
(Matthew 4:1-11)

**SOME PEOPLE ARE BOUND
BY A DEMON SPIRIT OF INFIRMITY**
Cast out the spirits with a word.
(Luke 13:11-13 / Mark 9:25 / Matthew 8:16)

**DEMONS AND SICKNESS ARE
SUBJECT TO THE NAME OF YESHUA**
*Lord, even the demons are subject (submit) to us in
your name.*
(Luke 10:17)

**THE NAME YESHUA IS ABOVE
THE NAMES OF SICKNESS OR PAIN**
*God exalted him and gave him a name above every
name.*
(Philippians 2:9)

**COMMAND SICKNESS OR PAIN
TO 'GO AWAY' IN JESUS' NAME**
*Whoever shall say and not doubt … shall have
what he says.*
(Mark 11:23)

**YOU DO NOT HAVE TO TAKE
SICKNESS OR DISEASE OR PAIN**
*He (Yeshua) took our infirmities, and carried away
our diseases.*
(Matthew 8:17)

**YOU CAN BE HEALED BY SAYING
GOD'S WORD AND BELIEVING IT**
*Confess with your mouth ... and believe in your
heart.*
(Romans 10:9)

**YOU CAN BE HEALED BY HEARING
OR READING GOD'S WORD**
He sent his word and healed them.
(Psalm 107:20)

**YOU CAN BE HEALED BY HANDS
LAID ON YOU IN JESUS' NAME**
*(Believers) shall lay hands on the sick, and they
shall recover.*
(Mark 16:18)

**YOU CAN BE HEALED BY
THE ANOINTING WITH OIL**
*Is any(one) sick? ... call for the elders of the
church.*
(James 5:14-15)

**YOU CAN BE HEALED IN
BODY, MIND AND SPIRIT**
Heal me, O Lord, and I shall be healed.
(Jeremiah 17:14)

YOU CAN BE HEALED BY
PROPER MENTAL ATTITUDE & PRAYER
All things are possible to him that believes.
(Mark 9:23)

YOU CAN BE HEALED BY A
PRAYER CLOTH PLACED ON YOUR BODY
*The diseases left them, and the evil spirits went out
of them.*
(Acts 19:11-12)

If you would like an anointed prayer cloth

sent to you to place on your body, write to:

WORLD SERVICES
P.O. Box 1001
Bonsall, CA 92003
USA

~ CHAPTER FORTY-TWO ~

HEALING FROM HEADACHES

JAW AND HEAD PAIN

DESCRIPTION

There are many types of headaches, including the most serious: Migraines. The purpose of this podcast is to lead you on a path to help you find relief ... and deliverance—total and permanent healing—from unnecessary pain and discomfort in the head and jaw.

The *World Health Organization* estimates that nearly half of the adult population suffers from headaches.[1]

One of the most insidious—but considered by many non-threatening—areas of disease is that which encompasses head pain, including jaw pain. It may be called disease because it is just that: "**dis**–ease, or "lack of ease, or "non–ease."

God wants YOU healed, healthy and whole. My job is to help you attain that position.

First, let's start with the problem. **Are you having either periodic or recurring pain in your head or jaw?** If it is constant (not just recurring or periodic) then you need a help NOW: you need a miracle or you need to see a doctor or call 911. First, let me PRAY for you.

> *"Father in Heaven, in the name of Your Son I command the pain to leave this person immediately ... NOW ... and I loose the HEALING POWER of Messiah Jesus to enter this person. Be healed and made whole in the Name of the LORD."*

Now ... it is time for YOU to pray. First, ask the LORD Jesus Christ to forgive your sins and to take over your life. Ask Messiah Jesus to be your LORD.

Next, if for some reason (known or unknown) you do NOT experience the release of pain—then if the problem has been either recurring or periodic—I want you to **plan a strategy** and ask God to guide you in this strategy. Do the following: Pray, and ask God to lead you to the following (they must be honest professionals with good reviews and references):

- A medical doctor (Primary Care Physician);

- A dentist;

- An ENT (Ear, Nose and Throat specialist); and,

- A chiropractor.

The Primary Care Physician (PCP) can check you and give you referrals to #2, #3, and #4 above. The dentist (#2) and the EEN (#3) and the Chiropractor (#4) can help you eliminate the source (or sources) of your problem. The dentist can identify if a condition in your teeth or gums is causing your head or jaw pain. The EEN can identify if a condition in your ears, nose or throat is causing the problem. The chiropractor can analyze your musculoskeletal system to identify if perhaps it is a subluxation complex problem causing your pain.

Because the vertebrae protect the spinal cord, even a small disturbance to the vertebrae can profoundly affect delicate nerve tissue. Also, the impairment to the nerve system can cause tissues and organs throughout the body to function poorly.

You will want to PRAY at each step of the way and ask God to help the doctor analyze your specific problem with accuracy. For example, if both the dentist and the EEN specialist tell you that you should be experiencing NO problem (that is, the pain in head or jaw pain is NOT being caused by a condition in your teeth, gums, ear, nose or throat) then it is a fairly good probability that the problem lies with a spinal (including the neck) or jaw condition.

Even if you have some teeth that need working on (for example, cavities), an honest dentist will tell you if that is NOT causing your problem with head or jaw pain. They may even tell you to come back when you are experiencing severe pain (if you are not at the time you see them) to help them provide you with a more accurate diagnosis.

If it turns out that it is a problem with the jaw or jaw misalignment or TMJ, the chiropractor may be able to adjust the alignment or treat the musculoskeletal condition that is the culprit. It may take only one treatment (adjustment) or you may need a successive number of treatments. **Restoring musculoskeletal**

balance is KEY to preventing and treating your headaches.

The **strategy** outlined above is to help you eliminate what is NOT causing your problem so that you can focus on what IS causing your problem. Then, **with prayer and directed activity you can focus on healing the root of the problem: the cause of the symptoms!**

Be careful about online video exercises for problems with your jaw or problems with TMJ as you may aggravate the situation. If you have narrowed the problem to jaw condition, then ask a chiropractor or other holistic health professional what is a good healthy and preventive maintenance routine. Even then, if you experience aggravation, stop immediately.

If you have access to a swimming pool, periodic (daily or other) light swimming may bring much sought after relief. It helps to reduce both muscular tension and stress. Give it a try and see ... and remember to pray for healing while you are swimming. **Learn to work with God. He is for you!** If you are Spirit-filled, pray in tongues while you are swimming.

Chiropractic can effectively relieve the most common types of headache: migraine (one-sided); tension type (vice like); and, cervicogenic (stemming from the neck). Abnormal motion of the neck joints can lead to headaches. Headaches can have one or more causes: biomechanical, vascular, psychological, genetic, neurological or environmental. Also, there are several possible headache triggers: excessive stress, chocolate, red wine, caffeine, aged cheeses, MSG, improper sleep patterns, weather changes, pollution, and vigorous or unbalanced exercise.

Regardless of the root cause, God wants you healed and healthy. And then ... you can go help others to healing and to a life of health! Pray right now and ask God to reveal the sources of your headaches—your jaw or head pain—and to heal you: either miraculously or to lead you in planning a strategy for healing. Remember, **it doesn't matter HOW God works ... just so He works!**

My personal medical PCP that I had for years used to tell me, **"God heals and doctors get the credit."**

For more info on healing and health, study the book, *Health and Healing Complete Guide to Wholeness.*

FOOTNOTE:

1. I personally believe that statistics supporting this statement by the *World Health Organization* are possibly skewed. As an international traveler to third world countries I can tell you that many headache problems in economically sub-standard geographic areas are due to associated problems such as malnutrition, bad health and tooth and gum disease. – *Prince Handley*

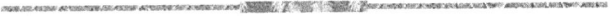

~ CHAPTER FORTY-THREE ~
HEALING FROM BACK PAIN

DESCRIPTION

There are many types, as well as causes, of back pain. Also, there are severities ranging from moderate to extreme ... and some, life threatening. Many people suffer for years with a condition that could have been taken care of in a short time ... and some, instantly. **God is the Healer and the Creator**—and by virtue of this fact —**He knows exactly what you need**.

There is nothing wrong with going to physicians or seeking medical help or advice.   But what we should do is seek the LORD first to see what He wants us to do. He may want to heal us by His sovereign power, over a period of time, or instantaneously.

There are many types, as well as causes of, back pain. There is neck pain, upper back pain, mid and lower back pain, and then the sacrum related conditions at the base of the spine. You have probably heard someone complain of sciatica which is caused by irritation of the nerve roots that lead to the sciatic nerve coming out of the spinal cord in the lower back. A bulging or ruptured disc is usually the primary culprit in such a condition. However, there can be other conditions involved.

Arthritis can cause bone spurs which can cause or exacerbate sciatica. Also, an injury can cause compression of the nerve roots. There are several other causes for sciatica, and the source of the irritation will usually dictate the treatment prescribed: physical therapy, medicine and sometimes surgery. Be very careful of exercise regimen with any type of back condtion, especially spinal related, as you could be aggravating the situation. Always check with your medical professional concerning any type of workouts, exercise and even stretching.

CAUTION: There is a condition known as Cauda Equina Syndrome which you might think is sciatica; however, it is very dangerous and without a MIRACLE from God may require urgent surgical treatment. Its symptoms can be similar to sciatica, and causes can be:

- A severe ruptured disk in the lumbar area (the most common cause).

- Narrowing of the spinal canal (stenosis).

- A spinal lesion or tumor.

- A spinal infection, inflammation, hemorrhage, or fracture.

- A complication from a severe lumbar spine injury such as a car crash, fall, gunshot, or stabbing.

- A birth defect such as an abnormal connection between blood vessels.

There are types of bone pain attributed to bone fusion or where the vertebrae grow over. One such condition is known as Ankylosing Spondylitis (AS). It affects the spine with pain and stiffness from the neck down to the lower back and does not necessarily confine itself to older people; **it happens most often to teenagers and men in their twenties**, and is characterized by stiffness from the neck down to the lower back, and can result in a rigid spine.

Back pain can be caused from injury, work, poor posture (sitting or standing), sports and recreation. But ... **the Good News is that YOU can be healed of back pain!** You may be thinking ... or saying ... *"I've had this condition for years!"* Well, let me tell you, my friend, that **Jesus, the Healer, has been healing for years!** There are some practical things you can do to help your situation:

- Exercise (check with a medical professional before starting an exercise or stretching regimen);

- Take proper nutrition and supplements;

- Get the required amount of sunshine (for Vitamin D);

- Rest your body and your mind.

Take advantage of physical helps like the "Teeter HangUps" inversion table. This helps reverse the effects of gravity and disc compression. (Check with your medical professional before using.)

The scope of this teaching is NOT to discuss specific types of therapy or treatments, but rather to present an alternative solution to problems that you or a loved one may be experiencing with back related issues. You can be healed today—NOW—by calling on the name of the LORD: **Who forgives all your sins, and Who heals all your diseases** (Psalm 103:3) The LORD's healing nature never changes. **It is God's will to heal you!**

Remember the lady in the Bible who was bent over for 18 years?

> *"And, behold, there was a woman which had a spirit of infirmity eighteen years, and was bowed together (bent over), and could not in anyway lift herself up.*
>
> *And when Jesus saw her, he called her to him, and said unto her, Woman, you are loosed from your infirmity.*
>
> *And he laid his hands on her: and immediately she was made straight, and glorified God."* (Matthew 13:11-13)

———————

MY TESTIMONIES

I am completely back pain FREE at this time in my life ... and I have been on Planet Earth for quite a while! My advice to you—*especially if you know the Great Physician, Messiah Jesus*—is: **NEVER GIVE UP!**

MY TESTIMONY # 1

Before I knew Jesus personally, I went for 13 years with terrible back pain. I don't know what caused it. I was a varsity wrestler in school, but I don't remember any happenings that would have caused (the devil's) pain. (I say "the devil's pain" because it was NOT **my** pain; it was pain the devil wanted me to have!) Also, I had been in NO serious accidents, not even small ones. By God's grace I have never had a broken bone in my lifetime. I have claimed the scripture for years (a prophetic one about Messiah Jesus' death on the cross) that says, *"He keeps all his bones; not one of them is broken."* (Psalm 34:20)

Here is how I was healed. My pain was so bad and so aggravating. I had been to a chiropractor years before and had learned or remembered how he had "fixed" my back to alleviate pain. So, I would lie on the floor and try to "fix" my back the way the chiropractor did.

I was miserable, and it got worse and worse! I was addicted to "cracking" my back. I probably was compounding the situation. It was such a miserable condition ... and, to make matters worse, at that time in my life I did NOT know about **the healing power of Christ!**

Finally, I began to wonder if the situation was NOT a physical problem, but possibly a "spirit" problem; in other words, a "spirit of affliction" sent by the devil to plague me while I was trying to do God's work! To give you an idea of how bad the situation was, if I were in a business environment where I had never been before, I would look to see if the receptionist stepped out of the office so I could lie on the floor and "crack" my back. I was miserable!

One day as I was on the floor ready to "crack" my back, **the Holy Spirit spoke to me.** He said, **"Why don't you let me take care of that for you?!"** Wow! I knew exactly what He meant. Instead of ME trying to fix the problem and compounding it each time I "cracked" my back, **the Holy Spirit wanted to FIX it.** It was such a temptation because when—and immediately after—I would "crack" my back, I would feel so much better ... until it started hurting again! I really had to resist "cracking" my back ... but realized at the same time, I didn't want to go through that all of my life. So ... I said, **"OK, Holy Spirit, I give this problem—this back condition—to You!"** That was it, it was over. PRAISE GOD! That was many years ago.

MY TESTIMONY #2

Another time—a different situation and condition—I experienced extreme pain in my upper right back below my shoulder. It was not a spinal problem, but **it would hurt so badly that I would cry**. I asked God different times to either heal me or take me home to Heaven! I went to medical doctors, I went to specialists, I went to physical therapy ... nothing worked. I even told two of the doctors I had that I asked the LORD, **"Either heal me or take me to Heaven,"** so they would know **how bad** the situation was.

Nothing worked! Finally, one night while travelling in another area of the country, before I went to bed, I prayed to God and said, **"Father, you can just send an Angel to touch me and I will be healed."** That night, while I was sleeping, **I was awakened with a loud "POP" in my back where the problem had been.** It was so loud it awakened me. **And I was perfectly healed.** I have never had that problem since, and never will. Thank God—it has been over 10 years—and thank the Holy Angel that God sent to touch me. Yes, "Touched by an Angel" has a special meaning to me!

PRAISE is also an important remedy for back pain.

- It lifts up and straightens the spinal column and relaxes it from a "stooped" condition. Learn to practice praise to God several times a day for at least 30 seconds.

- God lives in the praise of His people. *"But You are holy, O You that inhabits the praises of Israel."* (Psalm 22:3)

- The anointing breaks the yoke. Since God lives in the praise of His people, there is an anointing present with **true** praise, which can break an "assigned" attack on the body, mind or spirit. *"And it shall come to pass in that day, that **his burden***

215

shall be taken away from off thy shoulder, and his yoke from off thy neck, and the yoke shall be destroyed because of the anointing." (Isaiah 10:27)

■ Praise brings victory. King Jehoshaphat and the inhabitants of Judah and Jerusalem won a large battle utilizing praise. (Read 2 Chronicles Chapter 20, verses 1-30 in the Tanakh.)

CHECK THIS OUT: An Egyptian friend of mine, Magdy Girgis, was a member of our Board of Directors. He worked for Hughes Aircraft as did several Christians—who had been Baptized in the Holy Spirit—all of which spoke in tongues. They had Bible studies together every morning before work and also at lunch time. One day a man named Warren Meisenbach, who worked in the Engineering Department, came to their Bible study at lunch. Warren was NOT a believer and he asked them, *"What's this **born again** stuff you keep talking about?"* **Warren had been a "hunch back" for 15 years** (like the lady in the Bible I discussed earlier who had been bent over 18 years). Warren received Christ as his Lord that day, and asked the men to lay hands on him for healing. **Instantly ... they could hear his back "cracking' like: POP, POP, POP.** He **was perfectly straightened in a normal position.** When he went home his wife was dumbfounded because he was not only "straightened" but smiling for the first time in years! **Jesus is the Healer ... the Great Physician. Will you let Him heal YOU?**

If you want to meet the Healer—Jesus the Anointed One —NOW is the time! Invite God's Son, Jesus, to come into your life by praying **the following prayer**:

> *"Messiah Jesus, I know that you are The Great Physician. You loved me enough to shed your sinless blood and die for me on the cross stake that I might be healed.*
>
> *I know you are alive. Please forgive my sins, come into my life, and be my Master. Help me to live for you, and take me to Heaven when I die."*

I have selected two (2) books which will help you to **know how to deal with any type of pain**—so you can live PAIN FREE and serve God—and enjoy life the way God wants you to. Here they are:

Health and Healing Complete Guide to Wholeness

How to Receive God's Power with Gifts of the Spirit

The second book will help you know HOW to appropriate God's Power and to operate in the Gifts of the Holy Spirit.

ADDENDUM

I have seen many people healed by the LORD of back pain, back conditions and paralysis. I have witnessed many people walking out of their wheel chairs. I was holding a three day seminar at a church and I had asked the people present to join me in prayer and fasting for the last day as I was going to teach on healing. **A man was present who had been in a wheel chair for nine years due to two conditions**:

> **1**. A large 18 wheel semi-tractor truck had run into his automobile and he had five breaks in his spine; plus,

218

2. He had muscular dystrophy.

During Holy Communion he walked out of his wheel chair and never went back! Two years later, he gave his testimony in a large Presbyterian church and hundreds of people fell out of their seats under the Power of the Holy Spirit. **NEVER GIVE UP!**

~ CHAPTER FORTY-FOUR ~
HEALING THROUGH REST

One of the greatest means of healing today is simply by means of REST. You heard right: rest!

First of all, healing through rest is a promise provided for us in the Holy Bible. In the Tanakh, we read:

> "*If you keep your feet from stomping on the Sabbath—from pursuing your own interests on my holy day—if you call the Sabbath a delight and the LORD's Holy Day honorable; and if you honor it by not going your own ways and seeking your own pleasure or speaking merely idle words, then you will take delight in the Lord, and he will make you ride upon the high places of the earth; and he will make you feast on the inheritance of your ancestor Jacob, your father. Yes! The mouth of the Lord has spoken.*" – Isaiah 58:13-14

Notice, when you "**ride on the heights of the earth**" you have dominion ... you have perspective and are ABOVE the things of the earth. You are in a position of blessing by God. **You are blessed.** Also, when you **"feast on the inhertitance of you ancestor Jacob"** you are partaking spiritually—plus physically and materially—of the health and wealth of the father of the 12 tribes of Israel.

Notice something interesting. In the context of Isaiah Chapter 58 we read about fasting as well as rest. In my personal experience, one of the quickest ways to receive healing is through "fasting unto the LORD." Sometimes, just a three day fast with water only ... or, even a three day fast until 7 PM (and then eating healthy food) ... has brought immediate healing. Notice what God promises in Isaiah Chapter 58 concerning fasting: *"Then your light will break forth like the dawn, and **your healing will spring up quickly**; and your vindication will go before you, and the glory of the Lord will guard your back. Then you'll call, and the Lord will answer; you'll cry for help, and He will respond, 'I am here.'"* – Verses 8 and 9

Let me give you a personal testimony of how God used REST to bring me healing. I had been very busy holding evangelistic and tent meetings and in addition I had contracted for a busy schedule of radio production. Quickly I was entered into the Intensive Care center of the hospital with **several unknown rare diseases.** I was placed into an isolation room where even **the nurse was NOT allowed to enter**. When the nurse was taking my information (she had to stand outside the door), she asked me, *"What is your date of birth."* I asked her, *"Which one do you want?"* She said, *"Do you mean that you have been born more than once?"* I said, *"Yes, when I came out of my mother's womb ... AND ... when I gave my life to Jesus Christ."* She answered, *"I know what you're talking about. My father is a minister; but **I have never experienced the new birth**."* (I don't remember if she received the LORD there or not.) Then she asked me, *"What is your address?"* I then told her, *"Heaven."*

The nurse came back in a few minutes and said, *"Where were you? The doctor came in to see you in your room and you were NOT there."* I said, *"I have NOT left."* Then I realized that I was on the other side of my bed on the ground praying and the doctor could not see me from where he stood at the door.

Anyway, as soon as I was placed in the isolation ward room, I placed my hands behind my head—and laying back—**I realized instantly WHY I was there**. In a moment, the LORD impressed on my mind the verse from Isaiah 30:15: *"In returning and **rest** you shall be* *saved; in quietness and in confidence shall be your strength: **and you would not.***"

I then realized I had been busy doing God's work holding tent and evangelistic meetings, working to support the ministry, and travelling ... but NOT taking my Day of Rest. When I realized this, I repented before the **LORD** and asked for His forgiveness. Instantly, I could tell that I had been healed.

My friend, truly God has given YOU a practical and effective—cost effective—means of healing: REST.

*"Take my yoke upon you, and learn of me; for I am meek and lowly in heart: and you shall find **rest** unto your souls."* – Jesus of Nazareth

*"In returning and **rest** you shall be saved; in quietness and in confidence shall be your strength."* – Isaiah 30:15

If you want to meet the Healer—Jesus the Anointed One—NOW is the time! Invite God's Son, Jesus, to come into your life by praying **the following prayer**:

"Messiah Jesus, I know that you are The Great Physician. You loved me enough to shed your

sinless blood and die for me on the cross stake that I might be healed.

I know you are alive. Please forgive my sins, come into my life, and be my Master. Help me to live for you, and take me to Heaven when I die."

ADDENDUM

I have seen many people healed by the LORD of pain and paralysis. I have witnessed many people walking out of their wheel chairs.

I saw a lady who was so eaten up with cancer—she was in a wheel chair attended by her nurse—but **when the Holy spirit came upon her she stood up healed, walking out of her wheel chair**. She was so skinny from the affliction of cancer that when when stood up her petty coat (her slip undergarment) fell off to the ground.

I witnessed a man who had his head "locked" (positioned in a fixed relationship to his spine) into his wheel chair due to a spinal condition—if his head moved it would have caused serious trauma—and possibly death. **His nurse brought him to the service** and **when the Spirit**

of God breathed on him, the nurse "unlocked" his head and he walked out of the wheel chair healed.

I was holding a three day seminar at a church and I had asked the people present to join me in prayer and fasting for the last day as I was going to teach on healing. **A man was present who had been in a wheel chair for nine years due to two conditions:**

1. A large 18 wheel semi-tractor truck had run into his automobile and he had five breaks in his spine; plus,

2. He had muscular dystrophy for nine years. **During the Holy Communion he walked out of his wheel chair and never went back!** Two years later, he gave his testimony in a large Presbyterian church and hundreds of people fell out of their seats under the Power of the Holy Spirit. **NEVER GIVE UP!**

~ *CHAPTER FORTY-FIVE* ~
BONUS
SCRIPTURES FOR HEALING

DESCRIPTION

The Word of God builds faith for healing, is a channel for healing, a repository for healing, and an instrument for healing. Listen to it, read it, keep it in your heart. It is LIFE and HEALTH to your whole body.

I want to talk to you in this Bonus chapter about "**Scriptures for Healing**."

There is nothing like God's Word.

- It builds **faith** for healing.

- It is a **channel** for healing.

- It is a **repository** of healing.

- It is an **instrument** of healing.

In short, **God's Word heals!**

Proverbs 4:20-22 tells us:

> *"My son, attend to my words. Turn your ear to my sayings.*
>
> *Let them not depart from your eyes. Keep them in the midst of your heart.*
>
> *For they are **life** to those who find them, And **health** to their **whole body**."*

I'm going to share with you several healing Scriptures, but realize **it is God talking to you through His Promises**.

Torah: Exodus 15:26

> *"If thou wilt diligently hearken to the voice of the LORD your God, and will do that which is right in his sight, and will give ear to his commandments, and keep all his statutes, I will put none of these diseases upon you, which I have brought upon the Egyptians: for I am the LORD that heals you."*

Psalm 103:2-5

"Bless the LORD, O my soul, and forget not all his benefits:

Who forgives all your iniquities; who heals all thy diseases;

Who redeems your life from destruction; who crowns you with loving kindness and tender mercies; Who satisfies your mouth with good things; so that your youth is renewed like the eagle's."

Psalm 91:3, 5-6, 10

"For he will deliver you from the snare of the fowler, And from the deadly pestilence.

You shall not be afraid of the terror by night, nor of the arrow (weapon) that flies by day;

Nor of the plague or disease that walks in darkness, nor of the destruction that wastes at noonday.

No evil shall happen to you, neither shall any plague come near your dwelling."

Exodus 23:25

"And you shall serve the LORD your God, and he shall bless your bread, and your water; and I will take sickness away from the midst of you."

Psalm 41:4

"I said, LORD, be merciful unto me: heal my soul; for I have sinned against you."

Jeremiah 33:6

"Behold, I will bring it health and cure, and I will cure them, and will reveal unto them the abundance of peace and truth."

Isaiah 53:5

"But he was wounded for our transgressions, he was bruised for our iniquities: the chastisement of our peace was upon him; and with his stripes we are healed."

1 Peter 2:24

> *"Who his own self bare our sins in his own body on the tree, that we, being dead to sins, should live unto righteousness: by whose stripes you were healed."*

3 John 2

> *"Beloved, I wish above all things that you may prosper and be in health, even as your soul prospers."*

Psalm 107:20

> *"He sent his word, and healed them, and delivered them from their destructions."*

Matthew 9:35

> *"And Jesus went about all the cities and villages, teaching in their synagogues, and preaching the gospel of the kingdom, and healing every sickness and every disease among the people."*

Psalm 30:2

"O LORD my God, I cried unto you, and you have healed me."

Jeremiah 17:14

"Heal me, O LORD, and I will be healed; save me, and I will be saved: for you are my praise."

ADDENDUM TO BONUS

Remember, the Holy Bible tells us: *"So then faith comes by hearing, and hearing by the word of God."*

This is God's Word, settled in Heaven: a never changing fact concerning God's character; and **don't let anyone beat you out of His Will**. Don't let anyone—a minister, a rabbi, another person that claims they know Jesus—don't let them tell you that God does NOT keep His promises.

An article entitled, ***"Patient Knows Best,"*** appeared in the August 1991 issue of *The Reader's Digest.*

"A person's answer to the question, 'Is your health excellent, good, fair, or poor?' is a remarkable predictor of who will live or die over the next four years according to new findings.

*A study of more than 2800 men and women 65 and older found that **those who rate their health 'poor' are four to five times more likely to die in the next four years than those who rate their health 'excellent.'** This was the case even if examinations show the respondents to be in comparable health."*

A review of **five other large studies, totaling 23,000 people, showed similar conclusions**.

Combine your faith with God's Word. Do NOT lean on your circumstances; lean on God. Do NOT reinforce your conditions (sickness, disease, pain) by agreeing with them and talking about them. Talk to yourself the PROMISES of God. **The neural center of your brain knows how to transfer your faith words (God's promises) to your mental and physical conditions**.

My friend, the Messiah of Israel, Jesus, is the SAME: yesterday, today, and forever. (Hebrews 13:8) And, during His earthly ministry, **Jesus never refused healing to anyone!** And, my friend, **He wants to heal you right now.** The POWER of the Holy Spirit is upon you right now. Receive that MIRACLE you need in the name of Messiah Jesus!

✝

Call on Him today, my friend, and He will heal you and save you.

OTHER BOOKS BY PRINCE HANDLEY

Map of the End Times
How to Do Great Works
Flow Chart of Revelation
Action Keys for Success
Health and Healing Complete Guide to Wholeness
Prophetic Calendar for Israel & the Nations: Thru 2023
Healing Deliverance
How to Receive God's Power with Gifts of the Spirit
Healing for Mental and Physical Abuse
Victory Over Opposition and Resistance
Healing of Emotional Wounds
How to Be Healed and Live in Divine Health
Healing from Fear, Shame and Anger
How to Receive Healing and Bring Healing to Others
New Global Strategy: Enabling Missions
The Art of Christian Warfare
Success Cycles and Secrets
New Testament Bible Studies (A Study Manual)
Babylon the Bitch: Enemy of Israel
Resurrection Multiplication: Miracle Production
Faith and Quantum Physics: Your Future
Conflict Healing: Relational Health
Decision Making 101: Know for Sure
Total Person Toolbox
Prophecy, Transition & Miracles
Enhanced Humans: Mystery Matrix
Israel and Middle East: Past ~ Present ~ Future
Anarchy and revolution: A Prophecy
Real Miracles for Normal People
Sexual Immorality: Addiction of Loss
Healing Toolbox Plus: A to Z Workshop
Anointed Strategies: Power Plays

AVAILABLE AT AMAZON AND OTHER BOOK STORES

UNIVERSITY OF EXCELLENCE PRESS
San Diego ▪ London ▪ Tel Aviv

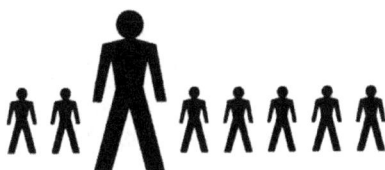

LIVE A LIFE OF EXCELLENCE

Email for seminars to:
princehandley@gmail.com

UNIVERSITY OF EXCELLENCE PRESS
San Diego ◼ London ◼ Tel Aviv

╬

NOTE

We listen to our readers. Tell us what **new** subject matter you would like to see published. Email your ideas to: universityofexcellence@gmail.com

LEGAL DISCLAIMER

The information in this book is not intended or implied to be a substitute for professional medical advice, diagnosis or treatment. All content—including text and information—contained in or available through this book or referred sources is for general information purposes only. Author Prince Handley, University of Excellence Press and/or Handley World Services Incorporated make no representation and assume no responsibility for the accuracy of information contained in or available through this book or referred sources, and such information is subject to change without notice. You are encouraged to confirm any information obtained from or through this book with other sources, and review all information regarding any medical condition or treatment with your physician.

Never disregard professional medical advice or delay seeking medical treatment because of something you have read in or accessed in this book or referred sources.

www.ingramcontent.com/pod-product-compliance
Lightning Source LLC
Chambersburg PA
CBHW050113280326
41933CB00010B/1081